Makeup Tutorial Book for Teens and Beginners

Essential Techniques, Tips, and Transformations for Aspiring Artists

C.Smith

Chapter 1: Introduction to Makeup 1
Welcome to the World of Makeup! 1
Chapter 2: A Brief History of Makeup 2
Importance of Makeup in Personal Grooming 6
Chapter 3: Importance of Makeup in Personal Grooming 8
Makeup as a Tool for Self-Expression and Confidence 8
Professional and Social Perceptions 9
The Transformative Power of Makeup 10
Inclusivity and Accessibility in Makeup 12
Makeup as a Skill and Art Form 13
Health and Skin Care Considerations 14
Chapter 4: Understanding Your Skin Type 17
The Foundation of Effective Makeup Application 17
Identifying Your Skin Type 18
The Importance of Understanding Your Skin Type 19
How to Determine Your Skin Type 21
Considerations for Changing Skin Types 22
Professional Consultation 23
Chapter 5: Basic Makeup Tools and Products 25
Essential Tools for Beginners 25
Guide to Choosing Your First Makeup Products 25
How to Read Makeup Labels 27
Chapter 6: Skin Care Basics 30
Daily Skin Care Routine for Healthy Skin 30
Importance of Sun Protection 31
Dealing with Common Teen Skin Issues 33
Chapter 7: Foundation and Concealer Techniques 35
Choosing the Right Shade 35
Application Tips for a Natural Look 36
How to Cover Blemishes and Under-Eye Circles 38
Chapter 8: Eye Makeup Essentials 40
Basic Eyeshadow Application 40
Eyeliner Techniques for Beginners 41
Mascara Tips for Full Lashes 43
Chapter 9: Brow Shaping and Filling 45
Finding Your Perfect Brow Shape 45
Tools for Brow Grooming 46
Filling and Defining Brows 47
Chapter 10: Blush and Contouring Basics 50
Choosing Blush for Your Skin Tone 50
Simple Contouring Techniques for Beginners 51
Highlighting Basics 52

Chapter 11: Lip Makeup **54**
   How to Choose Lip Colors 54
   Application Tips for Lipstick and Gloss 55
   Caring for Your Lips 56

Chapter 12: Everyday Makeup Looks **59**
   School-Friendly Makeup 59
   Natural Look Tutorial 60
   Makeup for Special Occasions 61

Chapter 13: Mastering Diverse Makeup Styles - Tutorials for Every Look **64**
   Quick and Easy Everyday Makeup Routine 64
   E-girl Makeup Tutorial 64
   Step-by-Step "Sun-Kissed" Glowy Makeup Tutorial 66
   Dewy Glass Skin Makeup Tutorial 75
   Glitter Eye Makeup Tutorial 77
   Easy Everyday Eyeshadow Makeup Tutorial 79
   Glossy Lips Makeup for Teens 80
   Graphic Eyeliner Makeup Tutorial 81
   Eyeliner Tutorial for Beginners 82
   Bold Eyebrow Tutorial 83
   Everyday Eye Makeup Tutorial 84
   Natural Glam Teenager Makeup Tutorial 86
   Teen Makeup Tutorial for Beginners 87

Chapter 14: Advanced Techniques - Elevating Your Makeup Mastery **90**
   Smokey Eye Tutorial 90
   Contouring and Highlighting Like a Pro 92
   Bold Lip Makeup Looks 94

Chapter 15: Makeup Hygiene and Maintenance **97**
   Cleaning Your Makeup Tools 97
   When to Replace Makeup Products 98
   Storing Your Makeup Correctly 99

Chapter 16: Ethical and Sustainable Makeup Choices **102**
   Understanding Cruelty-Free and Vegan Makeup 102
   Eco-Friendly Makeup Brands and Products 102
   Making Responsible Makeup Choices 102

Conclusion: Embracing Your Makeup Journey **104**
   Recap of Key Makeup Skills 104
   Encouragement for Your Personal Makeup Journey 104

Chapter 1: Introduction to Makeup

Welcome to the World of Makeup!

Embark on a fascinating journey into the realm of beauty and creativity, where the canvas is your own face and the paints are the myriad makeup products waiting to be explored. In this vibrant world, every brush stroke, every color choice, and every technique you learn is a step towards mastering an art form that is as ancient as civilization itself.

Makeup, in its essence, is a celebration of individuality and a tool for self-expression. It has the power to transform, not just in the physical sense, but in how we perceive and present ourselves. From the subtle enhancement of your natural features to the bold statements of artistic expression, makeup offers a unique platform for showcasing your personality.

But beyond the surface, makeup is also deeply intertwined with history and culture. It has been a constant companion of humanity, evolving through the ages, reflecting societal norms, and often, challenging them. From the dramatic kohl-lined eyes of ancient Egypt to the minimalist trends of the modern world, each era's makeup style tells a story of the people and the times.

Understanding your skin type is the first step in this journey. Whether your skin is dry, oily, combination, or sensitive, there is makeup out there that's perfect for you. Knowing your skin helps in selecting products that not only enhance your beauty but also nourish and protect your skin.

In the professional world, makeup can be a subtle yet powerful tool. It can convey professionalism, attention to detail, and a sense of personal pride. In personal settings, it's an outlet for creativity, a way to stand out, or blend in, depending on your mood and the occasion.

As you turn each page, remember that the world of makeup is as diverse as it is beautiful. It's a world that encourages experimentation, values diversity, and celebrates individual beauty. Whether you're a beginner or an enthusiast, there's always something new to learn, a different perspective to consider, and a fresh look to try.

So, welcome to this colorful world! May your journey through these pages inspire you, boost your confidence, and add a little extra sparkle to your everyday life. Let's dive in and discover the magic of makeup together.

Chapter 2: A Brief History of Makeup

Embarking on a journey through the history of makeup is like wandering through a vast, colorful gallery, where each era's styles and preferences reflect the societal values and technological advancements of the time. This exploration is not just about colors and trends; it's a narrative of human culture, rituals, and the ever-evolving definition of beauty.

The Dawn of Makeup

- The origins of makeup trace back to ancient civilizations. In Ancient Egypt, both men and women adorned their eyes with kohl, a practice rooted in both aesthetic and practical purposes, as it was believed to ward off evil spirits and reduce the glare of the sun.
- The use of natural pigments for body and face painting was common in many indigenous cultures around the world, serving purposes ranging from spiritual rituals to wartime markings.

Classical Antiquity

- In Ancient Greece and Rome, makeup began to signify social status. Pale skin was highly valued, often achieved using powders made from lead or chalk. This era also saw the use of natural dyes for lip and cheek staining, highlighting the human fascination with enhancing natural features.
- However, makeup was not without its critics. Philosophers and scholars often associated it with deceit and moral ambiguity, reflecting the societal tensions around the concept of beauty.

The Middle Ages and Renaissance

The Middle Ages: A Time of Subdued Beauty

- The Middle Ages, often characterized by its religious conservatism, saw a significant retreat from the ostentatious use of makeup that was prevalent in earlier times. This era, stretching approximately from the 5th to the late 15th century, was marked by a societal shift that viewed overt beauty enhancements with suspicion and sometimes, outright condemnation.
- Beauty ideals in medieval Europe were heavily influenced by the church, which often preached modesty and humility. Pale skin was still in vogue, symbolizing purity and nobility, a stark contrast to the laboring classes who were tanned from working outdoors. Women sometimes achieved this look using natural ingredients like lead or vinegar, but the application was far more restrained compared to earlier and later periods.
- The use of makeup was not entirely absent, however. Subtle enhancements like rosy cheeks and tinted lips were achieved using natural dyes from plants

and fruits. These practices, though minimal, laid the groundwork for the resurgence of makeup in the following era.

The Renaissance: A Rebirth of Beauty and Art

- The Renaissance, a period of great cultural, artistic, and political revival from the 14th to the 17th century, marked a dramatic shift in the world of makeup and beauty. This era, beginning in Italy and spreading across Europe, saw a renewed interest in the arts, science, and the human form.
- Makeup and cosmetics, reflecting the Renaissance's indulgence in beauty and art, became more elaborate and widespread. The pale skin trend continued, with both men and women seeking a porcelain-like complexion, a challenging endeavor during an era without modern sunscreens. Lead-based powders were commonly used, despite their dangerous side effects, to achieve this look.
- The Renaissance also saw the introduction of other cosmetic enhancements. Women began to pluck their hairlines to achieve a higher forehead, a trend influenced by portraits of esteemed beauties of the time. Kohl was used to darken eyelashes and eyebrows, and lips were often reddened with substances like cochineal, a dye derived from insects.
- Queen Elizabeth I of England became an iconic figure in Renaissance beauty. Her heavily made-up appearance, with a stark white face and bright red lips, set a standard for beauty that was emulated by the nobility of Europe. This look, however, was not without its perils; the lead-based makeup used by the Queen and her contemporaries led to serious skin and health problems.
- The Renaissance period was not just about following trends set by royalty; it was also a time of exploration and experimentation in cosmetics. Recipes for homemade cosmetics began to circulate, with ingredients ranging from natural dyes to more exotic substances like mercury and sulfur.

The Intersection of Beauty and Health

- The Middle Ages and Renaissance were pivotal in shaping the future of makeup and cosmetics. However, this period also highlighted the often-overlooked aspect of health in the pursuit of beauty. The use of toxic substances in makeup would continue for centuries, sparking a dialogue about the safety and regulation of cosmetic products that is still relevant today.

As we reflect on this era's impact on the history of makeup, it's clear that the Middle Ages and Renaissance were not just times of subdued beauty and artistic revival; they were periods that set the stage for the complex relationship between beauty, health, and societal norms that continues to evolve in the modern world of cosmetics.

The 17th and 18th Centuries

- Makeup became a tool of both genders in the European aristocracy. The 17th century's Baroque period favored dramatic looks, while the 18th century's Rococo period leaned towards more delicate, refined aesthetics.

- This era also witnessed the darker side of makeup, with toxic ingredients causing health problems, leading to a growing awareness and eventual shift towards safer cosmetics.

The 19th and 20th Centuries

- The Victorian era saw a return to a more natural look, with makeup being associated with immorality. However, the late 19th and early 20th centuries marked the beginning of the modern cosmetics industry, thanks to pioneers like Max Factor and Elizabeth Arden.
- The 20th century was a revolutionary period for makeup. The roaring 1920s introduced bold eye makeup and lipsticks, the 1960s celebrated dramatic eyes and pale lips, and the late 20th century saw an explosion of color and creativity.

The Modern Era: A Revolution in the World of Makeup

The Early 20th Century: The Birth of the Cosmetics Industry

- The dawn of the 20th century marked a pivotal moment in the history of makeup with the birth of the modern cosmetics industry. This era witnessed the transition from homemade recipes to commercially produced makeup, making beauty products more accessible to a broader audience. Icons like Max Factor and Elizabeth Arden were instrumental in popularizing makeup, not just as a tool for stage actors but for every woman.
- The 1920s, known as the Roaring Twenties, ushered in a dramatic change in makeup styles. Women began to assert their independence and rebellion against traditional norms, reflected in the bold, dramatic makeup of the time. Dark eyes, long lashes, and the iconic red lip became symbols of the modern woman.

Mid-20th Century: Evolution and Diversification

- Each subsequent decade brought its own unique styles. The 1950s emphasized glamour, with icons like Marilyn Monroe and Audrey Hepburn setting trends. The 1960s saw the emergence of the mod look, characterized by pale lipstick and heavy eyeliner, epitomized by models like Twiggy.
- The 1970s and 80s were eras of bold experimentation. Makeup became a way to make a statement, with vibrant colors, glitter, and a return to more natural looks coexisting in the cultural landscape. These decades also saw the rise of makeup for men, challenging traditional gender norms.

Late 20th Century to Early 21st Century: Technological Advancements and Inclusivity

- The late 20th and early 21st centuries witnessed significant technological advancements in makeup production. The development of new materials and techniques led to a wider variety of textures, finishes, and colors, allowing for more personalization and creativity in makeup application.

- This era also marked a shift towards inclusivity and diversity in the beauty industry. Brands began to recognize the need for products that cater to a diverse range of skin tones and types. Foundations and concealers in an extensive array of shades became available, challenging the industry's previous one-size-fits-all approach.

The Impact of Social Media and Global Influences

- The advent of social media in the 21st century revolutionized the way makeup is perceived and consumed. Platforms like YouTube, Instagram, and TikTok became spaces for makeup enthusiasts and professionals to share tips, tutorials, and diverse beauty standards. Influencers and beauty bloggers emerged as new authorities in beauty trends, democratizing and diversifying the industry.
- Global influences became more pronounced, with trends and techniques from Asia, Africa, and other regions gaining prominence. K-beauty (Korean beauty) and J-beauty (Japanese beauty), known for their innovative products and emphasis on skin health, became global phenomena.

Ethical and Sustainable Practices

- Recent years have also seen a growing awareness of ethical and sustainable practices in the makeup industry. Cruelty-free and vegan makeup products gained popularity, responding to consumer demand for ethical production. Brands also started focusing on sustainable packaging and environmentally friendly ingredients, reflecting a broader societal shift towards sustainability.

Looking to the Future

- The modern era of makeup is characterized by its rapid evolution, inclusivity, and adaptability to technological and societal changes. As we look to the future, the trends and practices of this era suggest a continued expansion of the definition of beauty, an ongoing commitment to inclusivity and sustainability, and an unwavering fascination with the transformative power of makeup.

The history of makeup, from its ancient rituals to the vibrant trends of modern days, is a compelling narrative of humanity's unending quest for beauty, self-expression, and individuality. It's a rich tapestry that vividly illustrates how our perceptions of beauty are deeply influenced by the culture, technology, and the evolving times we inhabit.

In the modern era, the story of makeup is characterized by its remarkable trajectory of continuous innovation and democratization. This journey began with the flapper girls of the 1920s, who, with their bold eyes and iconic red lips, signaled a new era of female empowerment and self-expression. These early trends set the stage for the dynamic and transformative role that makeup would continue to play throughout the 20th and into the 21st century.

As we progressed through the decades, each period marked its own unique contribution to the world of cosmetics. The mid-century brought glamorous icons and the bold experimentation of the 70s and 80s, while the turn of the century introduced technological advancements that transformed makeup into an even more versatile and inclusive tool. This era also witnessed the rise of social media, which further democratized beauty standards and practices, allowing for a global exchange of ideas, techniques, and trends. Influencers and digital platforms have since become integral to the industry, shaping and reflecting the ever-changing cultural shifts and beauty ideals.

The modern narrative of makeup also places significant emphasis on ethical and sustainable practices. With a growing consciousness towards the impact of beauty products on both the environment and animal welfare, the industry has seen a shift towards cruelty-free, vegan, and environmentally friendly products. This shift reflects a broader societal movement towards sustainability and ethical consumerism, further enriching the story of makeup with new values and principles.

Today, makeup stands not just as a tool for personal expression but as a dynamic and inclusive art form. It celebrates diversity and creativity in all its forms, embracing a wide array of styles, techniques, and products that cater to an ever-expanding spectrum of beauty ideals. The future of makeup, much like its past, is set to continue pushing the boundaries of creativity and inclusivity, ensuring that it remains a vibrant and integral part of our cultural and personal identities. This ongoing evolution of makeup is a testament to its enduring power and relevance, encapsulating humanity's endless pursuit of beauty and self-expression through the ages.

Importance of Makeup in Personal Grooming

Makeup as a Tool for Self-Expression and Confidence

- Makeup is much more than a mere beauty tool; it's a powerful medium for self-expression and personal empowerment. It allows individuals to showcase their personality, mood, and style in unique ways. Whether it's a subtle enhancement of natural features or a bold, artistic statement, makeup can significantly boost self-confidence and self-esteem. By mastering the art of makeup, one can learn to accentuate their best features, express their individuality, and face the world with greater assurance.

Professional and Social Perceptions

- In professional and social settings, makeup can play a crucial role in how individuals are perceived. A well-applied makeup look can convey professionalism, attention to detail, and a sense of preparedness. In many professional environments, makeup is considered an extension of grooming, akin to dressing appropriately for work. It can also be a form of respect in certain social situations, showing that one has taken the time to present themselves thoughtfully.

The Transformative Power of Makeup

- The transformative aspect of makeup is not just about physical appearance but also about the emotional and psychological impact. The process of applying makeup can be therapeutic, providing a time for self-care and relaxation. For many, it's a ritual that helps them prepare mentally and emotionally for the day ahead. The transformation that makeup can bring about is not just in one's look but also in their mindset and attitude.

Inclusivity and Accessibility in Makeup

- The modern era of makeup has seen a significant shift towards inclusivity and accessibility. Makeup is no longer seen as a one-size-fits-all solution but rather as a diverse array of products catering to all skin tones, types, and genders. This inclusive approach has democratized beauty, allowing more people to find products that suit their needs and express their identity. It's a recognition that beauty is diverse and that personal grooming through makeup should be accessible to everyone.

Makeup as a Skill and Art Form

- Applying makeup is both a skill and an art form. It requires understanding of color theory, textures, and techniques. Learning to apply makeup effectively is akin to learning any other skill – it takes practice, patience, and creativity. The artistry involved in makeup application allows for endless creativity and experimentation, making it an enjoyable and fulfilling practice.

Health and Skin Care Considerations

- Integral to the use of makeup in personal grooming is the understanding of its impact on skin health. Quality makeup products, when chosen correctly and used in moderation, can protect the skin and even offer benefits like sun protection. It's important to balance makeup use with good skin care practices, ensuring that skin is well-cared for and healthy.

In conclusion, makeup's role in personal grooming extends far beyond mere aesthetics. It's a multifaceted tool that can enhance confidence, influence perceptions, and provide a creative outlet for self-expression. The importance of makeup in personal grooming lies not just in its ability to beautify but also in its power to transform, empower, and provide a means for individual expression in our daily lives.

Chapter 3: Importance of Makeup in Personal Grooming

Makeup as a Tool for Self-Expression and Confidence

Enhancing Identity and Personal Style

Makeup is a profound tool for self-expression, offering individuals the ability to portray their inner selves through their outward appearance. It allows for the manifestation of personal style and identity in a tangible, visible way. By choosing colors, textures, and techniques that resonate with their personality, individuals use makeup to communicate who they are or who they aspire to be. This expression can range from the dramatic and avant-garde to the subtle and understated, adapting to the mood, occasion, and individual preferences.

Boosting Confidence and Self-Esteem

The impact of makeup on confidence and self-esteem cannot be overstated. For many, the application of makeup is a transformative experience that not only alters their physical appearance but also elevates their mental state. It can act as an armor or a comforting routine that prepares them to face the world. The confidence gained from knowing they look their best can be empowering, enhancing their ability to engage socially, perform professionally, and approach challenges with a positive mindset.

Creative Expression and Artistry

Makeup is an art form, and its application is a creative process. Each face is a unique canvas, and makeup is the medium with which diverse and imaginative looks are crafted. This creative process allows for exploration and experimentation, where traditional beauty norms can be challenged, and unique aesthetics can be explored. The artistry involved in makeup application provides a sense of achievement and satisfaction, further boosting self-confidence and providing an outlet for creative energy.

Emotional and Psychological Benefits

The routine of applying makeup often serves as a meditative and therapeutic practice. This personal time can be a moment of self-care and relaxation, allowing for reflection and mindfulness. The ritualistic nature of the makeup routine can provide a sense of stability and control, contributing positively to mental health. It's a daily act of self-love and affirmation, reinforcing a positive self-image and attitude.

Social Empowerment and Asserting Identity

In social contexts, makeup can be a powerful tool for asserting identity and gaining empowerment. It allows individuals to align their appearance with their identity, which can be particularly significant for those exploring their gender identity or expressing their cultural heritage. In this way, makeup becomes a form of communication and a declaration of self, offering a way to connect with others while celebrating individuality.

Adapting to Life's Various Roles and Situations

Makeup's versatility allows individuals to adapt their appearance to various roles and situations in their lives. Whether it's presenting a professional face in a business meeting, a glamorous look for a social event, or a bold statement for a creative endeavor, makeup can help to align an individual's external appearance with the specific context and their intended role within it.

In essence, makeup is much more than a cosmetic tool; it's a means of personal empowerment and self-expression. It offers a way to enhance not just physical beauty but also to bolster psychological well-being, express creativity, and navigate the diverse roles and situations of everyday life with confidence. As a dynamic and versatile medium, makeup empowers individuals to present themselves to the world in a way that is true to their identity and aspirations.

Professional and Social Perceptions

Makeup as a Reflection of Professionalism

In the professional sphere, makeup can be a subtle yet powerful tool. It's not merely about looking attractive but about presenting a polished and put-together image. In many work environments, makeup is seen as part of overall grooming and professionalism, akin to wearing appropriate attire. A well-applied, subtle makeup look can convey attention to detail, preparedness, and a sense of seriousness about one's role. For example, a light, neat makeup application can enhance features softly, suggesting a meticulous and conscientious attitude.

Influence on Social Interactions and First Impressions

Socially, makeup can significantly influence first impressions. The way we present ourselves, including our use of makeup, can affect how we are perceived by others. A bright lipstick or a carefully done eye makeup can be conversation starters and express a sense of confidence. Makeup can also be tailored to suit different social settings – a more vibrant look for a party or a subdued, natural look for a casual meet-up, each adapted to fit the social context and desired impression.

Cultural Norms and Expectations

Makeup's role in professional and social settings is also deeply influenced by cultural norms and expectations. In some cultures, makeup is expected and considered a basic aspect of grooming, especially in formal and professional scenarios. In others, it might be reserved for special occasions. Understanding and navigating these cultural nuances is crucial, as it reflects respect for social norms and an awareness of the diversity in attitudes towards makeup.

Empowerment and Self-Representation

Beyond conforming to norms, makeup can also be an empowering tool for self-representation. It allows individuals to project an image that aligns with their professional and social identities. In professional networking or social gatherings, the way one chooses to wear makeup can be a form of self-expression, showcasing aspects of their personality, creativity, and professional acumen.

Gender Dynamics and Makeup

The use of makeup in professional and social contexts also intersects with gender dynamics. Historically seen as a feminine practice, the growing acceptance of makeup across all genders challenges traditional gender norms. For many, makeup is a way to express their identity beyond gender stereotypes, contributing to a more inclusive understanding of beauty and grooming.

Balancing Authenticity and Expectations

Navigating the use of makeup in professional and social settings often involves balancing personal authenticity with societal expectations. While it's important to adhere to professional standards, it's equally important to remain true to one's sense of self. This balance can empower individuals to use makeup not as a mask, but as a tool to enhance their natural features and express their unique personality in a way that is respectful of the professional and social context.

In conclusion, the role of makeup in professional and social perceptions is multifaceted and significant. It extends beyond aesthetics, acting as a medium for communication, a reflection of cultural norms, and a tool for personal empowerment. In both professional and social realms, makeup can play a crucial role in how individuals are perceived, how they express themselves, and how they navigate the complex interplay of personal identity and societal expectations.

The Transformative Power of Makeup

Physical Transformation and Self-Perception

The most immediate impact of makeup is its ability to transform physical appearance. Even minimal makeup can enhance features, conceal imperfections, and bring out a person's best qualities. This physical transformation often leads to a shift in self-perception. When individuals feel that they look their best, it can substantially boost their self-esteem and confidence. This psychological shift is significant, as it can influence how they interact with the world around them.

Emotional and Psychological Impact

Applying makeup can be more than a routine; it's an act of self-care that offers emotional and psychological benefits. For many, the process is a therapeutic ritual that allows them to take time for themselves. It can be a period of creativity, relaxation, and meditation, providing a calming start to the day or a soothing transition to an evening out. The act of focusing on oneself, even for a short time, can be a powerful antidote to stress and a busy lifestyle.

Makeup as a Form of Artistic Expression

Beyond its cosmetic use, makeup is a form of artistic expression. It allows individuals to experiment with different looks, play with colors and textures, and express their moods and personalities. This form of creativity is empowering, as it enables people to see themselves in new ways and often discover aspects of their personality they hadn't explored before.

Social and Cultural Significance

Makeup also has significant social and cultural implications. It can be a tool for conforming to or rebelling against societal norms and expectations. In certain cultures, makeup is an integral part of traditional attire, carrying deep historical and cultural significance. In contemporary society, it can be a way to stand out, fit in, or make a statement about one's identity and beliefs.

Inclusivity and Representation

The modern beauty industry's focus on inclusivity has expanded the transformative power of makeup. With a wider range of shades and products suitable for all skin types, ethnicities, and genders, more people can use makeup to represent their true selves. This inclusivity in makeup means that individuals from all walks of life can find products that suit their needs, allowing them to express their identity confidently.

The Role of Makeup in Life Transitions

Makeup often accompanies individuals through various life stages and transitions. For instance, it can be a rite of passage for teenagers exploring their identity, a confidence booster for a job interview, or a means of embracing new phases of life, such as marriage or motherhood. In each of these scenarios, makeup serves as a companion in transformation, marking new beginnings and celebrating changes.

In summary, the transformative power of makeup extends far beyond surface-level changes. It influences self-perception, offers emotional and psychological benefits, serves as a medium for artistic expression, and plays a significant role in social and cultural contexts. As an inclusive tool for expression and empowerment, makeup is not just about altering appearances; it's about enabling individuals to present the best version of themselves to the world and, in doing so, transform their perception of themselves and how they are perceived by others.

Inclusivity and Accessibility in Makeup

Breaking Down Beauty Barriers

The modern makeup industry has made significant strides in promoting inclusivity and accessibility, breaking down the traditional barriers that once defined beauty standards. This shift is characterized by a broader representation of diverse skin tones, genders, ages, and cultural backgrounds. Makeup brands are increasingly recognizing the importance of catering to a diverse customer base, ensuring that everyone has access to products that suit their specific needs and preferences.

Expanding Shade Ranges and Product Diversity

One of the most notable changes in the makeup industry is the expansion of shade ranges in foundations, concealers, and other complexion products. Brands are now offering an extensive array of shades to accommodate the full spectrum of skin tones. This inclusivity ensures that individuals, regardless of their skin color, can find products that match and enhance their natural complexion.

Addressing Diverse Skin Types and Concerns

Beyond color, inclusivity in makeup also involves creating products for diverse skin types and concerns. Brands are formulating products suitable for sensitive skin, acne-prone skin, mature skin, and everything in between. This attention to diverse skin needs allows individuals to use makeup that not only enhances their appearance but also cares for their specific skin conditions.

Gender Inclusivity in the Beauty Industry

The beauty industry is also embracing gender inclusivity, moving away from the traditional view of makeup as a female-only domain. Makeup lines targeted at men and non-binary individuals are on the rise, challenging the gender norms and making the world of makeup more welcoming and inclusive for everyone, regardless of gender identity.

Accessibility for All Abilities

Accessibility in makeup also extends to individuals with disabilities. Brands are innovating with user-friendly packaging, easy-to-handle applicators, and tools designed for those with limited mobility or dexterity. These developments make it easier for everyone to enjoy the art of makeup, regardless of physical limitations.

Affordability and Economic Accessibility

Economic accessibility is another important aspect of inclusivity in makeup. High-quality makeup should not be a luxury reserved for a few. More brands are offering affordable options without compromising on quality, ensuring that individuals from all economic backgrounds can enjoy makeup.

Cultural Representation and Sensitivity

Inclusivity also means being culturally sensitive and representative. This involves respecting and celebrating cultural makeup traditions and ensuring that products and marketing campaigns are respectful and inclusive of different cultural backgrounds.

The Impact of Social Media and Community Feedback

Social media has played a pivotal role in driving the inclusivity movement in the beauty industry. Consumers now have a platform to voice their needs and critiques, pushing brands towards greater inclusivity. The makeup community online has become a powerful force in shaping industry trends and standards, emphasizing the need for representation and accessibility.

In conclusion, inclusivity and accessibility in makeup are about much more than expanding product ranges. It's about creating a beauty industry that welcomes and celebrates all individuals, regardless of their skin color, gender, age, ability, or economic status. This ongoing evolution towards a more inclusive and accessible makeup industry not only enriches the market with diverse products but also fosters a beauty culture that is respectful, representative, and empowering for everyone.

Makeup as a Skill and Art Form

The Artistry of Makeup

Makeup is not just a routine; it's a form of art. Like any artistic endeavor, it requires creativity, precision, and an understanding of color, texture, and form. Makeup artists are akin to painters; their canvas is the human face, and their medium is a diverse palette of cosmetics. This art form allows for the expression of mood, personality, and style, transcending traditional boundaries of art by being both ephemeral and personal.

Learning and Mastering Techniques

The skill of applying makeup is learned and honed over time. It involves mastering various techniques such as blending, contouring, highlighting, and shading. Each technique serves a specific purpose, from defining facial features to creating optical illusions of depth and dimension. The learning process is continuous and ever-evolving, as new products and styles emerge in the beauty industry.

Understanding Color Theory and Textures

A key aspect of makeup artistry is understanding color theory. This knowledge helps in selecting shades that complement individual skin tones, eye colors, and hair colors. Additionally, the understanding of textures – matte, satin, shimmer, and gloss – is crucial in achieving desired effects. For instance, matte textures can create depth, while shimmers highlight features.

Creativity and Personal Expression

Makeup is a powerful medium for personal expression. It allows individuals to experiment with their looks, try new trends, or even create their own unique styles. From theatrical makeup to everyday wear, the possibilities are limitless. This creative freedom not only enhances personal style but also encourages self-exploration and confidence.

Cultural and Historical Influences

The art of makeup is deeply influenced by cultural and historical contexts. Over the centuries, makeup styles have evolved, reflecting the social, cultural, and fashion trends of the time. Understanding these influences can add depth and meaning to the practice of makeup artistry, connecting the present with the rich history of beauty and adornment.

Professional Makeup Artistry

For those who pursue makeup as a career, professional artistry involves more than just application skills. It encompasses an understanding of facial anatomy, skin science, and the ability to work with diverse clients. Professional makeup artists must be adept at translating a client's vision into reality, whether for a wedding, a photoshoot, or a fashion show.

Innovation and Experimentation

The field of makeup encourages innovation and experimentation. Artists constantly explore new materials, techniques, and ideas, pushing the boundaries of traditional makeup. This exploration keeps the art form dynamic and exciting, ensuring that it continues to evolve and inspire.

In conclusion, makeup as a skill and art form is a complex and rewarding practice. It blends creativity, technical skill, and personal expression, offering a unique way to explore and present one's identity. Whether for personal enjoyment or professional pursuit, makeup artistry is a profound and fulfilling form of artistic expression, continuously enriched by the diverse experiences and creativity of those who practice it.

Health and Skin Care Considerations

Understanding the Impact of Makeup on Skin Health

When incorporating makeup into personal grooming, it's essential to consider its impact on skin health. The skin, being the largest organ of the body, can be affected by the types of products applied to it. Selecting makeup that complements and does not harm the skin is crucial. This means being mindful of ingredients, understanding your skin type, and choosing products that align with your skin's needs.

Choosing the Right Products for Your Skin Type

One of the keys to maintaining healthy skin while using makeup is to choose products suitable for your skin type. For instance, individuals with oily skin may benefit from non-comedogenic and oil-free products, while those with dry skin might look for hydrating and moisturizing makeup formulas. Those with sensitive skin should seek hypoallergenic options to minimize the risk of irritation.

The Importance of Quality and Safe Ingredients

The quality and safety of makeup ingredients are paramount. It's advisable to avoid products with harmful chemicals, such as parabens, phthalates, and synthetic fragrances, which can cause skin irritation, allergies, or long-term health issues. Instead, opting for makeup with natural, non-toxic ingredients can be beneficial for both skin health and overall wellness.

Balancing Makeup Use with Good Skin Care Habits

Regular and thorough makeup removal is essential for maintaining skin health. Sleeping with makeup on can clog pores, leading to breakouts and premature aging. A consistent nighttime skincare routine, including gentle cleansing to remove makeup, followed by moisturizing, can help preserve the skin's health and vitality.

The Role of Sun Protection

Sun protection should not be overlooked, even when wearing makeup. Many makeup products now include SPF, but it's important to ensure adequate sun protection, either through makeup or separate sunscreen products. This protects the skin from harmful UV rays, preventing sun damage, and maintaining overall skin health.

Understanding the Need for Regular Breaks

Giving your skin a break from makeup occasionally can be beneficial. These breaks allow the skin to breathe and recover, especially if there are any signs of irritation or breakouts. It's an opportunity to focus on skincare treatments that nourish and rejuvenate the skin.

Regular Cleaning of Makeup Tools

The cleanliness of makeup tools is often an overlooked aspect of skin health. Brushes and sponges can harbor bacteria, which can lead to skin irritation or acne. Regular washing of these tools is essential to prevent the buildup of bacteria and ensure that they are safe to use on the skin.

Staying Informed About Product Recalls and Updates

Finally, staying informed about product recalls and safety updates is important. The makeup industry continuously evolves, and being aware of any changes, especially those related to health and safety, is beneficial for informed decision-making.

In conclusion, the role of makeup in personal grooming is both multifaceted and significant, extending far beyond mere aesthetics. While it undeniably has the power to enhance appearance and boost confidence, its true importance lies in its impact on skin health and overall wellbeing. By carefully choosing the right products, adhering to good skincare habits, and staying informed about the ingredients and tools used, individuals can fully enjoy the myriad benefits of makeup. This approach ensures that while embracing the transformative and empowering aspects of makeup, one does not compromise on maintaining healthy skin.

Moreover, makeup serves as a powerful tool for self-expression and personal empowerment. It allows individuals to influence perceptions, showcase their creativity, and express their unique identity. Whether it's used to create bold statements or to subtly enhance natural features, makeup provides an outlet for creativity and personal expression that is deeply intertwined with our daily lives.

The importance of makeup in personal grooming, therefore, encompasses its ability not just to beautify, but also to transform and empower. It's a testament to how makeup can be a positive force in our lives, enriching our self-expression, boosting our confidence, and contributing to our personal and professional personas. Ultimately, when used thoughtfully and responsibly, makeup becomes more than just a cosmetic product; it becomes a vital component of our personal grooming that celebrates and enhances our individuality.

Chapter 4: Understanding Your Skin Type

The Foundation of Effective Makeup Application

Essential Understanding for Optimal Results

The foundation of effective makeup application lies in a deep understanding of your skin's unique characteristics and needs. Just as an artist must know their canvas, a successful makeup application starts with an awareness of the skin type you are working with. This knowledge is crucial for choosing products and techniques that enhance your natural beauty without compromising skin health.

Tailoring Your Approach to Suit Your Skin

Each skin type presents its own set of challenges and advantages in makeup application. For example, makeup on oily skin needs to manage excess sebum and prevent shine, whereas makeup on dry skin should aim to hydrate and avoid emphasizing dry patches. By understanding your skin type, you can tailor your makeup routine to address these specific concerns, ensuring that your makeup not only looks good but also feels comfortable throughout the day.

Enhancing Your Natural Beauty

Effective makeup application isn't about masking your natural skin; it's about enhancing what you naturally have. This approach ensures that your makeup complements rather than overpowers your features. Whether it's selecting the right foundation formula, choosing complementary colors, or applying products in a way that accentuates your best features, understanding your skin lays the groundwork for a makeup look that is both beautiful and harmonious with your natural appearance.

Creating a Lasting Effect

Knowing your skin type also contributes to the longevity of your makeup. For instance, makeup that is tailored to oily skin will include steps to control oil and prevent the makeup from sliding off, while makeup for dry skin will focus on moisture retention for a lasting, hydrated look. This knowledge helps in selecting the right primers, setting powders, and setting sprays that work best with your skin type, ensuring that your makeup stays put and looks fresh for longer.

Preventing Skin Concerns

Another important aspect of understanding your skin type is the prevention of common skin concerns. Using the wrong makeup products can exacerbate issues like acne, dryness, or sensitivity. By choosing products that are appropriate for your skin type, you can avoid potential adverse reactions and maintain healthy, glowing skin.

The Role of Skincare in Makeup Application

Effective makeup application is not just about the makeup itself; it also involves good skincare. Preparing your skin with the right skincare routine can drastically improve the application and look of your makeup. For example, properly moisturized skin can provide a smoother canvas for foundation, while using an appropriate exfoliator can prevent makeup from clinging to dry patches.

In summary, the foundation of effective makeup application is built upon a thorough understanding of your skin type. This knowledge allows you to select the right products, employ suitable techniques, and integrate a complementary skincare routine, all of which are key to achieving a flawless makeup look that enhances your natural beauty and maintains the health of your skin.

Identifying Your Skin Type

The Key to Personalized Makeup and Skincare

Understanding and identifying your skin type is crucial for selecting the right makeup and skincare products. Each skin type has unique characteristics and needs different care. Here's how you can identify your skin type and understand its specific requirements:

1. **Normal Skin**
    - Characteristics: Normal skin is well-balanced, neither too oily nor too dry. It has a regular texture, few imperfections, and no severe sensitivities. The pores are barely visible, and the skin's surface is neither greasy nor flaky.
    - Makeup Tips: People with normal skin have the most versatility in makeup choices. They can experiment with various formulations without much concern about adverse reactions.

2. **Oily Skin**
    - Characteristics: Oily skin is characterized by excess sebum production, leading to a shiny complexion, enlarged pores, and a tendency toward acne and blackheads.
    - Makeup Tips: For oily skin, look for oil-free, non-comedogenic makeup to avoid clogging pores. Matte formulations are ideal as they help control shine throughout the day.

3. **Dry Skin**
    - Characteristics: Dry skin often feels tight and may have flaky patches. It can appear dull due to a lack of moisture and may have more visible lines.

- Makeup Tips: Hydrating and creamy makeup formulations work best for dry skin. Look for products that provide moisture and have a dewy finish to add a natural glow.

4. **Combination Skin**
    - Characteristics: Combination skin features two or more different skin types on the face, typically with the T-zone (forehead, nose, chin) being oily and the cheeks being normal or dry.
    - Makeup Tips: Combination skin may require using different products for different areas. For example, a mattifying primer for the T-zone and a hydrating foundation for the cheeks.

5. **Sensitive Skin**
    - Characteristics: Sensitive skin is prone to inflammation and irritation. It might react to certain ingredients, fragrances, or environmental factors more quickly than other skin types.
    - Makeup Tips: Choose hypoallergenic and fragrance-free makeup products to minimize the risk of irritation. It's also important to conduct patch tests before using new products.

Conducting a Skin Type Test

- A simple way to determine your skin type at home is the 'bare-faced method':
    1. Cleanse your face with a gentle cleanser to remove all traces of makeup or dirt.
    2. Pat your face dry and leave it bare (without applying any additional skincare products).
    3. After about an hour, examine your skin's texture and how it feels. Check for any shine on your forehead, nose, and chin (indicators of oily skin) and feel whether your cheeks are dry or tight (signs of dryness).
    4. If your skin feels comfortable and balanced, you likely have normal skin.

Adapting to Skin Changes

- Remember that skin type can change over time due to factors like age, hormonal fluctuations, or environmental changes. Regular assessment of your skin type can ensure that you are always using the most appropriate makeup and skincare products.

By identifying your skin type, you can tailor your makeup and skincare routine to suit your specific needs, leading to better overall skin health and more effective makeup application.

The Importance of Understanding Your Skin Type

Tailoring Your Makeup and Skincare Regimen

Recognizing and understanding your skin type is not just a trivial aspect of beauty care; it's a critical component for tailoring your makeup and skincare regimen. This knowledge directly influences the choice of products and techniques you use, ensuring they are effective and beneficial for your skin.

1. **Selecting Suitable Makeup Products**

    - **Right Foundation Match**: Your skin type determines the type of foundation that will look best. For example, matte foundations are typically suited for oily skin, while hydrating formulas are ideal for dry skin.
    - **Enhancing Wearability**: Makeup that complements your skin type tends to last longer and look more natural. Oily skin types benefit from long-wear, oil-controlling makeup, whereas dry skin requires products that prevent flaking and cakiness.
    - **Reducing Skin Problems**: Using makeup suited for your skin type can help minimize skin problems. For instance, non-comedogenic makeup is essential for acne-prone skin to prevent pore clogging.

2. **Effective Skin Care Routine**
    - **Targeted Care**: Understanding your skin type allows you to choose skincare products that address specific concerns effectively. Oily skin may need more astringents and lightweight moisturizers, while dry skin may require richer, more emollient creams.
    - **Preventing Irritation**: Especially for sensitive skin, using the right skincare products is crucial to prevent irritation or allergic reactions.

3. **Improved Skin Health**

    - **Long-term Benefits**: Using the correct products for your skin type contributes to overall skin health. It can prevent problems like excessive dryness, oiliness, acne, and sensitivity, leading to a more balanced and healthy complexion in the long run.
    - **Age Management**: Tailored skincare and makeup routines can also help in managing aging signs more effectively. For example, dry skin might need more nourishing anti-aging ingredients, while oily skin might focus on products with anti-acne properties.

4. **Personalized Beauty Experience**

    - **Enhanced Confidence**: When your makeup and skincare align with your skin type, you are likely to feel more confident and comfortable in

your skin. This leads to a more positive beauty experience and a feeling of well-being.
- **Creative Expression**: Understanding your skin type also opens up opportunities for more creative and effective makeup application, allowing you to experiment with different looks and techniques that suit your skin.

5. **Cost-Effectiveness**

    - **Wise Investments**: Knowing your skin type helps in making more informed choices when purchasing products. It prevents waste of money on unsuitable items and ensures that your investments in makeup and skincare are more likely to yield satisfactory results.

In essence, understanding your skin type is essential for a holistic approach to beauty. It's not just about enhancing appearance; it's about nurturing and maintaining the health and integrity of your skin. This understanding forms the basis of a personalized beauty routine that resonates with your skin's unique characteristics and needs, leading to better outcomes both aesthetically and health-wise.

How to Determine Your Skin Type

A Step-by-Step Guide

Determining your skin type is a crucial step in creating a tailored skincare and makeup routine. Here's a simple guide to help you understand your skin's characteristics:

1. **Start with a Clean Face**
    - Begin by gently cleansing your face with a mild cleanser to remove makeup, oil, and impurities. This step ensures that you're observing your skin's natural state, unaffected by any products you've previously applied.

2. **Wait and Observe**
    - After cleansing, don't apply any skincare products. Let your skin rest and return to its natural state. Wait for about an hour to allow your skin to demonstrate its natural characteristics. This waiting period is essential for observing how your skin behaves without any external influences.

3. **Check for Oiliness and Dryness**

- After an hour, examine your skin, particularly in the T-zone (forehead, nose, and chin), as well as the cheeks. Use a clean tissue to gently press on different areas of your face.
  - **Oily Skin**: If the tissue picks up oily spots from the T-zone and possibly other areas, you likely have oily skin. Oily skin often appears shiny and may feel greasy.
  - **Dry Skin**: If your skin feels tight, looks flaky, or the tissue shows little to no oil, you probably have dry skin. Dry skin often lacks visible pores and has a matte appearance.
  - **Combination Skin**: If the tissue reveals oil from the T-zone but not from your cheeks, your skin type is likely combination. Combination skin is characterized by an oily T-zone and normal to dry cheeks.
  - **Normal Skin**: If there are no signs of excess oil or dryness and your skin feels comfortable, you likely have normal skin. Normal skin is well-balanced, with few visible pores or imperfections.
  - **Sensitive Skin**: If you notice redness, itching, burning, or irritation during this process or in general, you may have sensitive skin. This skin type requires special care to avoid aggravation.

4. **Consider Other Factors**
   - Skin type isn't just about oiliness or dryness. Consider other factors like sensitivity, acne-prone areas, or signs of aging. These factors can influence the type of skincare and makeup products you choose.

5. **Note Environmental and Lifestyle Impacts**
   - Be aware that environmental factors (like humidity and temperature) and lifestyle choices (such as diet and stress levels) can affect your skin. Your skin type can change over time due to these influences, so it's good to reassess periodically.

6. **Consult a Professional**
   - If you're uncertain or if your skin has specific concerns, consulting a dermatologist or a skincare professional can provide you with more detailed insights. They can offer guidance tailored to your skin's unique needs.

By understanding your skin type, you can make more informed decisions about the products and care routines that will work best for you, leading to healthier skin and more effective makeup application. Remember, skin type can evolve, so it's beneficial to reassess your skin periodically to ensure that you're always giving it the care it needs.

Considerations for Changing Skin Types

Adapting to Your Skin's Evolving Needs

Your skin type is not a static aspect of your physiology; it can change over time due to various factors. Adapting your skincare and makeup routines to these changes is essential for maintaining healthy skin and effective makeup application. Here are key considerations to keep in mind:

1. **Age-Related Changes**
   - As you age, your skin undergoes natural changes. It tends to become drier and less elastic due to decreased oil production and collagen levels. Adjust your skincare to include more hydrating and anti-aging products. Makeup choices might also shift towards products that provide hydration and don't settle into fine lines.
2. **Hormonal Fluctuations**
   - Hormones play a significant role in skin behavior. Adolescence, pregnancy, menstrual cycles, and menopause can all cause changes in skin type. For example, you might experience increased oiliness and acne during hormonal fluctuations. Adapting your skincare routine to include oil-control and acne-fighting products during these times can be beneficial.
3. **Climate and Environmental Factors**
   - Your environment significantly affects your skin. High humidity can increase oiliness, while cold, dry weather can lead to dry and chapped skin. In humid climates, you might need to switch to lighter, oil-free products, whereas in colder climates, richer, more emollient products can help protect and hydrate your skin.
4. **Lifestyle and Diet**
   - Lifestyle choices, such as diet, stress levels, and smoking, can impact your skin. A balanced diet rich in antioxidants and staying hydrated can promote healthy skin. High stress can trigger breakouts or exacerbate skin conditions like eczema, making stress management and skincare that targets these issues important.
5. **Product Sensitivities and Allergic Reactions**
   - Over time, your skin may develop sensitivities or allergies to certain ingredients. Pay attention to how your skin reacts to different products. If irritation occurs, reevaluate your skincare and makeup to identify and eliminate potential irritants.
6. **Reassessment is Key**
   - Periodically reassess your skin type, especially when you notice changes in your skin's appearance or behavior. This reassessment will

ensure that you are always using products that cater to your current skin needs.
7. **Professional Guidance**
    - If you're noticing significant changes in your skin that are difficult to manage, it may be helpful to seek advice from a dermatologist. They can provide professional insights into your changing skin type and recommend appropriate products and treatments.

Understanding that your skin type can change over time is crucial in maintaining its health and appearance. By staying attuned to these changes and adapting your skincare and makeup routines accordingly, you can ensure that your skin receives the care it needs at every stage of life. This adaptability not only helps in addressing immediate skin concerns but also contributes to the long-term health and vitality of your skin.

Professional Consultation

Leveraging Expertise for Personalized Skin Care

While self-assessment of your skin type can be effective, there are times when professional consultation can be invaluable. Seeking advice from a dermatologist or a skincare professional offers several benefits, particularly for those with specific skin concerns or conditions. Here's why and when to consider a professional consultation:

1. **Expert Diagnosis**
    - Dermatologists are skilled in accurately diagnosing skin types and identifying underlying skin conditions. They can offer a more nuanced understanding of your skin's needs, which might not be apparent through self-assessment.
2. **Addressing Specific Skin Concerns**
    - If you're struggling with specific skin issues such as chronic acne, severe dryness, eczema, rosacea, or other skin conditions, a dermatologist can provide targeted treatments and product recommendations. These specialized treatments are often more effective than general over-the-counter products.
3. **Customized Skincare Regimen**
    - Professionals can help develop a customized skincare regimen that is tailored to your unique skin type, concerns, and goals. They can recommend the right combination of products and ingredients that work synergistically for optimal skin health.
4. **Guidance on Product Selection**
    - With the overwhelming array of skincare and makeup products available, choosing the right ones for your skin can be daunting. Dermatologists can guide you in selecting products that are effective

and suitable for your skin type, potentially saving you time and money spent on trial and error.

5. **Understanding Skin Reactions and Allergies**
   - If you've experienced adverse reactions, such as allergies or sensitivities, to certain skincare or makeup products, a professional can help pinpoint the causes and advise on safer alternatives.
6. **Staying Informed About Treatments and Trends**
   - Dermatologists stay abreast of the latest developments in skincare treatments and technologies. Consulting with them can provide access to advanced treatments and cutting-edge products that might not yet be widely available.
7. **Long-Term Skin Health**
   - Regular consultations with a skin professional can be integral to maintaining long-term skin health. They can help monitor changes in your skin over time and adjust your skincare regimen accordingly.
8. **When to Seek Professional Help**
   - Consider scheduling a consultation if you have persistent skin problems, are unsure about your skin type, have experienced negative reactions to products, or simply want to improve your overall skin health and appearance.

Incorporating professional consultation into your skincare journey adds an invaluable dimension of expertise and personalization. A dermatologist's guidance can elevate your skincare routine, address specific concerns effectively, and ensure that your skin receives the best possible care tailored to its unique needs.

In this chapter, we delve deeper into each skin type, offering tips and recommendations for makeup and skincare that will help you enhance your natural beauty while taking care of your skin's unique needs. Understanding your skin type is not just about better makeup application; it's about nurturing the health of your skin and embracing your natural beauty.

Chapter 5: Basic Makeup Tools and Products

Embarking on your makeup journey can be both exciting and overwhelming, given the plethora of tools and products available in the market. This chapter is designed to guide beginners through the essentials of makeup tools and products, helping you build a solid foundation for your makeup routine.

Essential Tools for Beginners

1. **Brushes and Applicators**
   - A set of basic brushes is crucial for applying makeup precisely and effectively. Key brushes include a foundation brush, a powder brush, an eyeshadow brush, a blending brush, and a blush brush.
   - Don't overlook the importance of a good sponge or beauty blender for seamless blending, especially for liquid and cream products.
2. **Eyelash Curler**
   - An eyelash curler can make a significant difference, especially if you have straight lashes. It helps to curl the lashes, making the eyes look wider and more awake.
3. **Tweezers**
   - A pair of tweezers is essential for grooming brows, removing stray hairs, and placing false lashes.
4. **Sharpener**
   - If you use pencil eyeliners or lip liners, a sharpener is a must-have for keeping your pencils in top condition.
5. **Mirror**
   - A good, clear mirror, preferably with magnification options, is vital for precise application.

Guide to Choosing Your First Makeup Products

Selecting your first set of makeup products can be a delightful yet daunting task. Here's a guide to help you make informed choices:

Foundation

- **Skin Tone Match**: The foundation should match your skin tone perfectly. Test several shades along your jawline, and check them in natural light. The right shade will blend seamlessly into your skin without leaving any lines of demarcation.
- **Skin Type Consideration**: Consider your skin type when choosing the formula. For oily skin, look for oil-free and mattifying foundations. For dry skin, hydrating and luminous finishes work best. If you have combination skin, a balance between matte and dewy formulations is ideal.

- **Coverage Level**: Decide on the coverage you need. Light coverage is great for a natural look, medium coverage is good for evening out skin tone, and full coverage is suitable for concealing significant blemishes or discoloration.

Concealer

- **Shade Selection**: A concealer used for hiding blemishes should match your foundation closely. For under-eye concealing, choose a shade that is one or two shades lighter than your foundation to brighten the area.
- **Formula**: Liquid concealers are versatile and work for most skin types. Stick or cream concealers offer more coverage and are ideal for spot-concealing.

Powder

- **Setting Powder**: A setting powder helps to set your foundation and concealer, reducing shine and prolonging the wear of your makeup. You can choose between loose powder, which offers a lighter, more natural finish, and pressed powder, which is more convenient for touch-ups.
- **Tinted vs. Translucent**: Tinted powders offer a bit of coverage and color, while translucent powders are invisible on the skin and suit all skin tones.

Basic Eye Makeup

- **Neutral Eyeshadow Palette**: A palette with neutral shades is versatile for both day and night looks. Look for a mix of matte and shimmer finishes to experiment with different styles.
- **Eyeliner**: A pencil eyeliner in black or brown is a good starting point. These colors are great for defining the eyes without being too harsh.
- **Mascara**: Choose a mascara that suits your needs, whether it's for lengthening, volumizing, or curling. Waterproof formulas are great for long wear but require a good makeup remover.

Blush and Bronzer

- **Blush**: A blush in pink, peach, or coral tones can add a healthy color to your cheeks. Cream blushes blend easily and are great for beginners.
- **Bronzer**: For subtle contouring and adding warmth, choose a bronzer one or two shades darker than your skin tone. Avoid anything too orange or glittery.

Lipstick or Lip Gloss

- **Shade Range**: Start with shades that you feel comfortable wearing. Nudes, pinks, corals, and light reds are versatile and beginner-friendly.
- **Formula**: Consider the finish - matte lipsticks offer longer wear but can be drying, while glosses add shine and hydration.

Makeup Remover

- **Gentle and Effective**: A good makeup remover is crucial for skin health. Opt for gentle, hydrating removers, especially if you wear waterproof or long-wear makeup.

In summary, when choosing your first makeup products, it's important to consider your skin type, your comfort level with different products, and the kind of look you wish to achieve. Start with the basics and gradually expand your collection as you become more comfortable with application techniques and discover what works best for you. Remember, makeup is a form of self-expression, and the most important thing is to have fun with it!

How to Read Makeup Labels

Understanding makeup labels is crucial for selecting products that are safe, effective, and suitable for your skin type and ethical preferences. Here's a breakdown of what to look for when reading makeup labels:

Ingredient List

- **Order of Ingredients**: The ingredients are listed in descending order of concentration. The first few ingredients usually make up the bulk of the product.
- **Key Ingredients**: Look for beneficial ingredients like hyaluronic acid for hydration, salicylic acid for acne-prone skin, and antioxidants like Vitamin C.
- **Potential Irritants**: Be aware of ingredients that might cause irritation or allergic reactions, especially if you have sensitive skin. Common irritants include certain alcohols, fragrances, and sulfates.
- **Comedogenic Ingredients**: If you're prone to acne, avoid ingredients that can clog pores (comedogenic), such as certain oils and silicones.

Expiration Date

- **Shelf Life**: The expiration date indicates how long the product is safe to use after opening. Using makeup beyond this date can lead to skin irritation, infections, and ineffective performance.
- **Period After Opening (PAO) Symbol**: This symbol looks like a little open jar with a number followed by "M", indicating the number of months the product is safe to use after opening.

Labels and Certifications

- **Non-Comedogenic**: Ideal for acne-prone skin as it indicates the product is formulated not to clog pores.

- **Hypoallergenic**: Suggests the product is less likely to cause allergic reactions, though it's not a guarantee.
- **Cruelty-Free and Vegan**: Cruelty-free products are not tested on animals, and vegan products do not contain animal-derived ingredients.
- **Organic or Natural**: Look for certifications like USDA Organic or ECOCERT for products claiming to be organic or natural.

SPF Content

- **Sun Protection Factor**: Makeup with SPF can provide additional sun protection, but it's often not enough on its own. For full protection, use a separate sunscreen, especially if the makeup has SPF lower than 30 or if you'll be in the sun for an extended period.

Shade Names and Numbers

- **Shade Matching**: Shade names and numbers can be confusing. Typically, "C" might stand for cool undertones, "N" for neutral, and "W" for warm. Numbers often indicate the depth of the shade.
- **Consistency Across Brands**: Be aware that shade names and numbers are not standardized across brands. Always test the product to ensure a proper match.

Patch Test Indication

- **Safety First**: Products, especially those with active ingredients like retinoids or acids, may recommend a patch test to ensure you don't have an adverse reaction.
- **Patch Test Method**: Apply a small amount of the product to a discreet area of your skin, like the inside of your wrist, and wait 24-48 hours to check for any reaction.

Additional Tips

- **Packaging Symbols**: Look for symbols like the open-flame symbol (indicating flammability) or the green dot (suggesting the packaging is recyclable).
- **Ingredient Research**: If you're unsure about an ingredient, do some research or consult a dermatologist, especially for ingredients high up on the list.

By understanding the nuances of makeup labels, you can make more informed decisions about the products you choose, ensuring they meet your skin care needs, makeup preferences, and ethical standards. This knowledge is not only essential for achieving the best results but also for maintaining the health and safety of your skin.

As we conclude this chapter on basic makeup tools and products, it's evident that the journey into the world of makeup is both exhilarating and enlightening. We've explored the essential tools that form the backbone of any makeup kit, from versatile brushes and applicators to practical items like tweezers and eyelash curlers. Each tool has its unique role in enhancing your beauty routine, providing the means to apply and perfect your makeup with precision and ease.

In selecting your first makeup products, we've delved into the essentials, guiding you through the process of choosing foundations, concealers, powders, and more. The key is to find products that not only match your skin tone and type but also align with your personal style and the looks you wish to achieve. Whether it's the natural subtlety of a neutral eyeshadow palette or the bold statement of a classic red lipstick, each product you choose adds a chapter to your unique beauty story.

Understanding makeup labels is another crucial aspect we've covered, equipping you with the knowledge to make informed choices about the products you use. From decoding ingredient lists to understanding the importance of expiration dates and SPF content, this knowledge ensures that your makeup choices are safe, effective, and in harmony with your skin's health and ethical standards.

As you embark on or continue your makeup journey, remember that these tools and products are not just about enhancing physical appearance; they are instruments of self-expression and creativity. Makeup is an ever-evolving art, and you are the artist. Your face is the canvas, and these tools and products are your palette and brushes. The looks you create can reflect your mood, showcase your personality, and even transform your perception of yourself.

In essence, the world of makeup is vast and varied, offering endless possibilities for exploration and expression. Whether you're a beginner just starting out or someone looking to refine their existing skills, the journey is personal and unique to each individual. Embrace it with enthusiasm, experiment with confidence, and most importantly, have fun with every brush stroke and color choice. Remember, in the art of makeup, you are the creator of your own beauty narrative.

Chapter 6: Skin Care Basics

The journey to beautiful makeup begins with the canvas of your skin. Proper skin care is essential for maintaining healthy, radiant skin and forms the foundation for any successful makeup application. In this chapter, we'll explore the fundamentals of skin care, focusing on daily routines, sun protection, and addressing common skin issues faced by teens.

Daily Skin Care Routine for Healthy Skin

A well-rounded daily skincare routine is essential for maintaining healthy, radiant skin. Each step, from cleansing to moisturizing, plays a vital role in skin health:

Cleansing

- **Purpose**: Cleansing is the first and fundamental step in any skincare routine. It removes dirt, oil, makeup, and environmental pollutants from the skin, preventing pore clogging and skin issues.
- **Choosing a Cleanser**: For oily or acne-prone skin, a gel-based or foaming cleanser with ingredients like salicylic acid can help control oil and fight acne. For dry or sensitive skin, creamy, hydrating cleansers with soothing ingredients like aloe vera or glycerin are recommended. Avoid harsh soaps and opt for pH-balanced products.
- **Double Cleansing**: Consider double cleansing in the evening, especially if you wear makeup. Start with an oil-based cleanser to dissolve makeup, followed by a water-based cleanser for a deeper clean.

Toning

- **Benefits**: Toners help to remove any last traces of impurities or makeup after cleansing. They also restore the skin's pH balance, which can be disrupted after cleansing, and provide an initial layer of hydration.
- **Choosing a Toner**: Look for alcohol-free toners that suit your skin type. Ingredients like witch hazel or tea tree oil are great for oily or acne-prone skin, while rosewater or chamomile are beneficial for dry or sensitive skin.
- **Application**: Apply toner gently with a cotton pad or with your hands, patting it onto the skin.

Moisturizing

- **Importance**: Moisturizers lock in hydration, protect the skin barrier, and prevent dryness. Even oily skin needs moisturization, as skipping this step can lead to overproduction of oil.
- **Selection**: For oily skin, choose light, oil-free, or gel-based moisturizers. For dry skin, richer creams with ingredients like hyaluronic acid or ceramides are ideal. For combination skin, you may need different types of moisturizers for different areas.

Exfoliating

- **Purpose**: Exfoliation removes dead skin cells from the skin's surface, promoting a brighter complexion and improving the effectiveness of other skincare products.
- **Types of Exfoliants**: There are two main types – physical exfoliants (scrubs) and chemical exfoliants (like AHAs and BHAs). Chemical exfoliants are generally preferred for their even and gentle exfoliation.
- **Frequency**: Over-exfoliating can damage the skin barrier, so limit this to once or twice a week, depending on your skin's tolerance.

Targeted Treatments

- **Addressing Specific Concerns**: Use serums or spot treatments to address specific issues like acne, pigmentation, or aging signs. Serums are concentrated formulas that target specific concerns with active ingredients.
- **Order of Application**: Apply these treatments after toning and before moisturizing, so the active ingredients can penetrate the skin effectively.

Consistency is Key

- **Routine Regularity**: Consistency is crucial in skincare. Adhering to your routine both morning and night ensures the best results.
- **Patience and Persistence**: Some products, especially those that target specific concerns like acne or hyperpigmentation, require time to show results. Be patient and give products several weeks to work.

Remember, the key to effective skincare lies in understanding your skin's unique needs and being consistent with your routine. Regular care with the right products will lead to healthier, more radiant skin, providing a perfect base for any makeup application.

Importance of Sun Protection

Daily Sunscreen Use

- **Crucial Defense Against UV Rays**: Sunscreen acts as a critical barrier between your skin and the sun's harmful ultraviolet (UV) rays. These rays are responsible for not only sunburns but also long-term damage such as premature aging, characterized by wrinkles, loss of skin elasticity, and age spots.
- **Broad-Spectrum Protection**: Opt for a broad-spectrum sunscreen, which offers protection against both UVA and UVB rays. UVA rays penetrate deeply into the skin, causing aging and long-term damage, while UVB rays cause sunburn.

- **SPF Recommendations**: The Sun Protection Factor (SPF) indicates the level of protection against UVB rays. Dermatologists recommend using a sunscreen with at least SPF 30, which blocks about 97% of UVB rays. Higher SPFs provide marginally more protection.
- **All-Weather Necessity**: UV rays can be damaging year-round and can penetrate through clouds and even glass. This means sunscreen is essential every day, whether it's sunny or overcast.
- **Correct Application**: Apply sunscreen liberally on all exposed areas of the skin, including the face, neck, ears, and hands. Remember that to achieve the SPF protection indicated on the label, a generous amount needs to be applied.

Reapplication

- **Maintaining Effective Protection**: Sunscreen should be reapplied every two hours, or more frequently if you're swimming, sweating, or towel-drying. Sunscreen can easily wash off or be removed, and its protective capabilities diminish over time.
- **Timing of Reapplication**: If you're using a chemical sunscreen (which absorbs UV rays), apply it at least 15 minutes before sun exposure. Physical sunscreens (which reflect UV rays) are effective immediately upon application.

Additional Protection

- **Protective Clothing**: Wear long-sleeved shirts, long pants, or long skirts to cover as much skin as possible. Fabrics with a tight weave offer better protection.
- **Hats and Sunglasses**: A wide-brimmed hat can provide shade and protect areas often exposed to the sun, like the ears, eyes, forehead, nose, and scalp. Sunglasses with UV protection are crucial for protecting your eyes and the delicate skin around them.
- **Seeking Shade**: When outdoors, especially between 10 a.m. and 4 p.m. when the sun's rays are strongest, seek shade whenever possible.
- **Sun Protective Factor (UPF) Clothing**: Consider wearing clothing with a UPF rating, which indicates how much UV radiation a fabric allows to reach your skin. A UPF 50 fabric blocks 98% of the sun's rays.

Understanding Sunscreen Ingredients

- **Chemical vs. Physical Sunscreens**: Chemical sunscreens contain organic compounds that absorb UV radiation, while physical sunscreens contain mineral ingredients like titanium dioxide or zinc oxide that reflect UV rays.
- **Sensitive Skin Considerations**: For sensitive skin, physical sunscreens are often recommended as they are less likely to cause irritation.

The Role of Sunscreen in Overall Health

- **Reducing Skin Cancer Risks**: Regular sunscreen use can significantly reduce the risk of developing skin cancers, including melanoma, the most dangerous form.
- **Preventative Health Measure**: Incorporating sunscreen into your daily routine is a preventative health measure that contributes to long-term skin health and overall well-being.

In summary, sun protection is an indispensable part of skincare. It goes beyond mere cosmetic concerns and plays a pivotal role in safeguarding your skin's health and preventing serious conditions like skin cancer. By incorporating daily sunscreen use, reapplication, and additional protective measures into your lifestyle, you actively contribute to maintaining the health and youthfulness of your skin.

Dealing with Common Teen Skin Issues

Adolescence brings about significant changes in the skin, often leading to various skin concerns. Understanding and properly addressing these issues can pave the way for healthier skin during the teen years and beyond.

Acne

- **Underlying Causes**: Hormonal fluctuations during teenage years can lead to increased oil production, contributing to acne. Factors like genetics, stress, and certain lifestyle choices can also play a role.
- **Skincare and Makeup**: Choose non-comedogenic (won't clog pores) and oil-free skincare and makeup products. Heavy, oily products can exacerbate acne.
- **Active Ingredients**: Look for products with benzoyl peroxide, which kills acne-causing bacteria, and salicylic acid, which helps unclog pores. Start with lower concentrations to gauge skin sensitivity.
- **Regular Cleansing**: Gently cleanse your face twice daily to remove excess oil and impurities. Avoid scrubbing harshly, as this can irritate the skin and worsen acne.
- **Avoid Picking and Popping**: Picking at acne can lead to scarring and further inflammation. Instead, use spot treatments for breakouts.

Oily Skin

- **Oil-Control Products**: Use products formulated for oily skin. These can help control excess shine and oil without overly drying the skin.
- **Gentle Cleansing**: Over-washing or using harsh cleansers can strip the skin of its natural oils, prompting increased oil production. Opt for gentle, pH-balanced cleansers.

- **Blotting Papers**: These can be used throughout the day to blot excess oil without stripping moisture from the skin.
- **Lightweight Moisturizers**: Hydration is still important for oily skin. Choose lightweight, water-based moisturizers that hydrate without adding excess oil.

Dry and Sensitive Skin

- **Hydrating Products**: Look for products rich in hydrating ingredients like hyaluronic acid, glycerin, and ceramides. These can help restore moisture and strengthen the skin barrier.
- **Gentle Exfoliation**: While exfoliation is important, avoid harsh scrubs. Instead, opt for mild chemical exfoliants, like lactic acid, used sparingly.
- **Avoid Irritants**: Steer clear of products with alcohol, fragrances, and other potential irritants that can exacerbate dryness and sensitivity.
- **Protective Barrier**: In colder months, protect your skin against harsh weather with richer creams and protective balms.

Lifestyle Factors

- **Diet and Hydration**: A balanced diet rich in fruits, vegetables, and whole grains can promote skin health. Staying hydrated is also key to maintaining healthy skin.
- **Stress Management**: High stress can trigger or worsen skin issues. Engaging in stress-reducing activities like exercise, meditation, or hobbies can positively impact your skin.
- **Sleep**: Adequate sleep is crucial for skin health. It allows the skin to repair and regenerate.

Consultation with Dermatologist

- **Professional Advice**: If over-the-counter products aren't effective, or if your skin issues are severe, a dermatologist can offer tailored advice and treatment options.
- **Prescription Treatments**: For persistent acne or other skin concerns, prescription treatments might be necessary. These can include topical retinoids, antibiotics, or other specialized medications.

Navigating the complexities of skin care, especially during the teenage years, is a journey that requires a harmonious blend of proper skin care practices, lifestyle adjustments, and at times, professional guidance. The key lies in understanding and responding to the unique needs of your skin, a process that allows for effective management of common skin issues often encountered during adolescence. By adopting a skincare routine that caters specifically to your individual skin type and concerns, you lay the groundwork for lifelong skin health. It's important to remember that every person's skin is unique, and a product or routine that works for one individual may not be as effective for another. Patience and persistence are crucial in exploring and finding the right balance for your skin's unique needs.

In essence, the fundamentals of effective skincare involve a deep understanding of your skin's characteristics and requirements. Establishing a consistent and thoughtful skincare routine is essential, and when this routine is combined with diligent sun protection and specific treatments for individual skin concerns, it leads to the development of healthy, radiant skin. This strong foundation of skincare not only enhances your natural beauty but also provides an ideal canvas for makeup application. Through these concerted efforts in skincare, you cultivate not only a routine but a lifelong practice that maintains and enhances the health and vitality of your skin.

Chapter 7: Foundation and Concealer Techniques

Mastering the application of foundation and concealer is essential for creating a flawless makeup look. These base products set the tone for your entire makeup routine, providing a smooth, even canvas. In this chapter, we'll explore how to choose the right shades of foundation and concealer, share tips for achieving a natural look, and discuss techniques to effectively cover blemishes and under-eye circles.

Choosing the Right Shade

Choosing the perfect foundation shade is crucial for a natural, flawless makeup look. It's about more than just matching your skin color; it involves understanding your skin's undertones, testing for the right match, and adapting to changes in your skin tone throughout the year.

Understanding Undertones

- **Significance of Undertones**: Your skin's undertone remains consistent regardless of changes in your skin color due to sun exposure or other factors. It's the underlying hue beneath the surface of your skin.
- **Determining Your Undertone**: One method to determine your undertone is to look at the veins on your wrist. If they appear blue or purple, you likely have cool undertones. If they look green, you have warm undertones. If it's hard to discern, you likely have neutral undertones.
- **Impact on Shade Selection**: Foundations are often categorized by undertones. Selecting a foundation that matches your undertone will ensure it complements your natural skin color and offers a more seamless match.

Shade Matching

- **Testing Foundation Shades**: The best place to test foundation is along your jawline. The ideal foundation shade should disappear into your skin, matching both your face and neck.
- **Natural Light Testing**: Always check your foundation shade in natural daylight. Artificial lighting can alter the appearance of the foundation, leading to an incorrect match.
- **Seeking Assistance**: Don't hesitate to ask for help at makeup counters. Professionals can assist in shade matching and often provide samples to try before purchasing.

Seasonal Changes

- **Adapting to Skin Tone Variations**: Your skin tone can vary with seasonal changes, particularly if you spend time outdoors. You might find your summer shade is too dark for the winter months or vice versa.

- **Having Multiple Shades**: Consider keeping two foundation shades in your makeup kit – one that matches your skin tone in the summer and another for the winter. You can also mix these shades during transitional periods for a custom match.
- **Adjusting with Bronzer or Highlighter**: If your foundation is slightly off due to seasonal changes, you can adjust the color with bronzer or highlighter. A bit of bronzer can warm up a foundation that's too light, while a highlighter can lighten a foundation that's a bit too dark.

Additional Tips

- **Sample Before Buying**: If possible, get a sample of the foundation to try at home. This allows you to test the foundation under different lighting conditions and ensure it works well with your other makeup products.
- **Consider Skin Type**: Be aware that your skin type can affect how the foundation appears on your skin. For instance, oilier skin can sometimes darken the foundation (known as oxidation), so you might need to choose a slightly lighter shade.

Choosing the right foundation shade is a blend of art and science. By understanding your undertones, meticulously testing shades, and being adaptable to changes in your skin tone, you can select a foundation that enhances your natural complexion beautifully. Remember, the goal is to find a shade that looks like your skin, only better.

Application Tips for a Natural Look

Creating a natural makeup look with foundation is about more than just applying the product; it's about preparing your skin properly, using the right tools, and employing techniques that enhance your natural beauty. In this comprehensive guide, we'll walk you through the steps to effortlessly achieve that flawless complexion you've been dreaming of.

Prepping the Skin

- **Cleanse and Moisturize**: Always start with clean skin. Use a gentle cleanser to remove any impurities or residue. Follow up with a moisturizer suited to your skin type. Well-hydrated skin ensures an even application and prevents the foundation from clinging to dry patches.
- **Primer Application**: A primer can significantly improve the longevity and appearance of your foundation. It smooths out pores, fine lines, and creates a seamless canvas. If you have oily skin, look for a mattifying primer. For dry skin, a hydrating primer works best.
- **Sunscreen**: If your foundation doesn't contain SPF, apply sunscreen before the primer. This step is crucial for protecting your skin from harmful UV rays.

Tools for Application

- **Makeup Sponge**: Dampen the sponge for a more sheer, dewy application. Bounce the sponge gently on your skin to blend the foundation. This tool is excellent for a buildable, airbrushed finish.
- **Foundation Brush**: A brush provides more precise application and fuller coverage. Use a flat brush for liquid foundations and a dense brush for powder foundations. Use downward strokes to apply and blend the product.
- **Fingers**: For those who prefer a minimalistic approach, fingers can be the perfect tool. They're great for warming up the product and providing a light, natural coverage. Be sure to wash your hands thoroughly before application.

Technique

- **Thin Layers**: Apply the foundation in thin, light layers. This approach prevents cakiness and gives you more control over the coverage. It's easier to add more product than to take it away.
- **Blending**: Start at the center of your face where most imperfections typically are and blend outwards. Ensure you blend well into your hairline, jawline, and neck to avoid visible lines. Pay attention to the edges and blend seamlessly.
- **Trouble Areas**: For areas that need more coverage, like under-eye circles or blemishes, gently tap a small amount of foundation or concealer with your finger or a small brush. Avoid rubbing as it can wipe the product away.

Setting the Foundation

- **Translucent Powder**: Use a light dusting of translucent powder to set your foundation. Focus on areas prone to oiliness, such as the T-zone. Translucent powder helps to reduce shine and set makeup without adding extra weight or color.
- **Powder Application**: Use a large, fluffy brush for a light application. Press and roll the brush onto the skin instead of sweeping to avoid disturbing the foundation underneath.
- **Avoid Over-Powdering**: Be cautious not to over-apply powder, as it can make your skin look dry and cakey. If you have dry skin, you might even skip this step or only powder specific areas.

By following these steps and techniques, you can achieve a natural-looking foundation application that enhances your complexion while maintaining the skin-like finish. The goal is to even out your skin tone and subtly perfect your skin without masking its natural beauty. Remember, the best foundation application is the one that looks like your skin at its best.

How to Cover Blemishes and Under-Eye Circles

Achieving a flawless makeup look often involves concealing imperfections like blemishes and under-eye circles. With the right techniques and products, you can effectively camouflage these areas for a smooth, even complexion. Here's a detailed guide on how to do just that:

Concealing Blemishes

- **Product Selection**: After applying your foundation, select a concealer that closely matches your skin tone for blemish coverage. The right concealer should blend seamlessly into your foundation.
- **Application Technique**: Use a small concealer brush or a clean fingertip for precise application. Gently dab the concealer onto the blemish. Avoid rubbing or dragging the skin, as this can remove both the concealer and the foundation underneath, reducing coverage.
- **Blending**: Softly blend the edges of the concealer into the surrounding skin to avoid a noticeable spot. The goal is to make the concealer indistinguishable from your foundation.
- **Layering**: If the blemish is still visible, wait for the first layer of concealer to set, then apply another thin layer. Layering in small amounts offers better coverage and looks more natural than applying a lot of product at once.

Under-Eye Circles

- **Shade Selection**: For under-eye circles, choose a concealer that is one or two shades lighter than your foundation. This will help to brighten the area.
- **Application Shape**: Apply the concealer in a triangular shape with the base along your lower lash line and the point extending towards the cheek. This technique not only covers dark circles but also illuminates and lifts the entire eye area.
- **Blending Method**: Gently blend the concealer using a damp sponge, a concealer brush, or your ring finger. The ring finger naturally applies less pressure, making it ideal for the delicate under-eye skin.

Setting Concealer

- **Preventing Creases**: To ensure your concealer stays in place and doesn't crease, especially in the under-eye area, set it with a light application of translucent powder.
- **Powder Application**: Use a small, fluffy brush to lightly dust the powder over the concealer. This will set the makeup and prolong its wear.

Using Color Correctors

- **Correcting Discoloration**: For more pronounced skin discoloration, such as dark circles or red spots, a color corrector can be very effective. These products use the principles of color theory to neutralize unwanted colors.
- **Corrector Shades**: Use peach or orange tones to counteract blue or purple under-eye circles. Green correctors are excellent for neutralizing redness in blemishes or rosacea.
- **Application Order**: Apply the color corrector before your concealer. Once the discoloration is neutralized with the corrector, you can apply the concealer as you would normally.

Mastering the art of foundation and concealer application is crucial for achieving a flawless makeup base. By honing these techniques, you can effectively conceal blemishes and under-eye circles, resulting in a smooth and even complexion. The secret to successful concealing lies in blending meticulously and selecting the appropriate colors to address your specific skin concerns. As you become accustomed to these methods, they will seamlessly integrate into your makeup routine, becoming both easy and effective. Remember, the journey to flawless makeup involves not just the right products and tools, but also the application techniques that best suit your skin type and coverage needs. With consistent practice and experimentation, you'll find the perfect approach that works for you, enhancing your natural beauty and elevating your makeup skills.

Chapter 8: Eye Makeup Essentials

Eye makeup can dramatically enhance your overall look, drawing attention to your eyes and expressing your personal style. In this chapter, we'll explore the basics of eye makeup, focusing on essential techniques for eye shadow application, eyeliner, and mascara. These foundational skills are key to creating a variety of eye makeup looks, from subtle and natural to bold and dramatic.

Basic Eyeshadow Application

Mastering the art of eyeshadow application can elevate your makeup look from simple to stunning. It's all about understanding the basics and then gradually building upon them. Here's an in-depth look at how to create beautiful eyeshadow looks.

Priming the Eyelids

- **Importance of Priming**: Eyeshadow primer is essential for creating a smooth canvas. It helps in evening out skin tone, ensuring that the eyeshadow adheres better and stays vibrant throughout the day without creasing or fading.
- **Alternatives to Primer**: If you don't have a specific eye primer, a small amount of concealer or foundation can also serve the purpose. They provide a neutral base and help in concealing any discoloration on the eyelids.

Choosing Colors

- **Neutral Palette for Beginners**: Start with neutral shades like beiges, browns, and soft pinks. These colors are versatile and less intimidating for beginners. They're great for creating a range of looks, from a subtle daytime appearance to a more defined evening look.
- **Understanding Color Theory**: Knowing which colors complement your eye color can enhance the overall impact. For instance, bronze and copper tones beautifully accentuate blue eyes, while purples and mauves make green eyes pop.

Basic Technique

- **Applying the Base Color**: Begin with a light, neutral color over your entire eyelid. This base shade evens out the skin tone on your eyelid and helps with blending subsequent colors.
- **Defining the Crease**: Use a slightly darker shade in the crease of your eye to add depth. This creates dimension, making your eyes stand out more. The key is to blend the crease color well, using a windshield wiper motion with a fluffy brush to avoid harsh lines.
- **Blending**: Blending is crucial in eyeshadow application. Ensure there are no visible lines between different shades. Blended eyeshadow gives a more professional and polished look.

Highlighting

- **Enhancing with Lighter Shades**: Apply a lighter, shimmery shade on the brow bone and the inner corner of your eyes. Highlighting these areas brings brightness to your eyes, making them appear larger and more awake.
- **Shimmer vs. Matte**: While shimmery eyeshadows are great for highlighting, matte shadows work well for the base and crease, especially in a professional or subtle makeup look.

Building Up

- **Adding More Colors**: Once you're comfortable with basic application, start experimenting with more colors. Adding a darker shade to the outer corner of your eye can intensify your look. You can also play with different textures, like metallics or glitters, for special occasions.
- **Layering and Blending**: Apply additional colors in layers, blending each one before adding another. This helps create a gradient effect where colors seamlessly blend into one another.

Additional Tips

- **Quality Brushes**: Invest in good-quality brushes for precise application and effective blending. Different brushes serve different purposes, like flat brushes for application and fluffy brushes for blending.
- **Practice and Experimentation**: Practice is key to perfecting your eyeshadow technique. Don't be afraid to experiment with different colors and styles to find what looks best on you.

Eyeshadow application is a fun and creative aspect of makeup. By starting with these basic techniques and gradually incorporating more complex elements, you can create stunning eye looks that enhance your natural beauty and complement your overall makeup style.

Eyeliner Techniques for Beginners

Eyeliner is a versatile tool in makeup, capable of transforming the look of your eyes dramatically. For beginners, mastering eyeliner application can be challenging, but with the right techniques and some practice, it can become an enjoyable part of your beauty routine. Here's a detailed look at various eyeliner techniques suited for those just starting out.

Pencil Eyeliner

- **Ease of Use**: Pencil eyeliners are ideal for beginners due to their ease of control and forgiveness in application. They allow for a more gradual and controlled line, making them perfect for everyday looks.

- **Basic Application**: Start by gently pulling your eyelid taut and drawing thin lines as close as possible to your lash line. This technique defines the eyes subtly.
- **Smudging for Effect**: One of the advantages of pencil liners is their blendability. For a softer, smoky eye look, apply the liner and then use a smudge brush or a cotton swab to softly blur the line.
- **Sharpening the Pencil**: Keep your eyeliner pencil well-sharpened for more precise lines, but if you prefer a smudged look, a slightly duller tip works better.

Liquid or Gel Eyeliner

- **Precision and Intensity**: Liquid and gel eyeliners provide a more dramatic and intense look. They are great for creating sharp, clean lines but require a steadier hand.
- **Application Tips**: When using liquid or gel liners, start with small strokes and slowly connect them. You can use a small, angled brush for gel liners for more precision.
- **Practicing Control**: Practice steady hand movements and control. Resting your elbow on a table while applying can help stabilize your hand.

Creating a Wing

- **The Winged Look**: Winged eyeliner is a classic look that elongates and lifts the eye. To create a wing, start by drawing a line from the outer corner of your eye, angling it upward towards the end of your eyebrow.
- **Connecting the Lines**: Extend this line back towards your lash line, creating a triangle on the outer corner of your eye. Fill in the triangle and then draw a line from the inner corner of your eye, connecting it to the wing.
- **Symmetry and Practice**: Achieving symmetry in both eyes can be challenging. Use small dots or dashes as guides before connecting them. Practice makes perfect, so don't be discouraged if it takes several tries to get it right.

Tightlining

- **Natural Enhancement**: Tightlining involves applying eyeliner right between the lashes on the upper waterline. This technique is excellent for making your lashes appear thicker and more voluminous without an obvious eyeliner look.
- **Technique**: Gently lift your upper lid and apply the eyeliner to the waterline. Pencil eyeliners are usually best for this technique. Be careful to avoid poking your eye and use short, gentle strokes.

Each of these techniques offers a different style and effect and mastering them can significantly enhance your eye makeup game. Start with the basics, like the pencil eyeliner, and gradually progress to more advanced techniques like liquid or gel eyeliners and winged looks. Remember, the key to perfect eyeliner is patience and practice. Over time, you'll develop a steady hand and discover the styles that best complement your eye shape and personal aesthetic.

Mascara Tips for Full Lashes

Mascara is a transformative makeup tool that can dramatically enhance your eyes by adding length, volume, and definition to your lashes. Here's a more detailed guide to help you maximize the impact of your mascara and achieve fuller, more captivating lashes.

Curling Lashes

- **Preparation for Mascara**: Curling your lashes is an essential step before applying mascara. It helps to lift and shape your lashes, creating a more open and awake look to your eyes.
- **Proper Technique**: Open the eyelash curler and place it at the base of your upper lashes. Gently clamp down near the roots and hold for a few seconds. You can repeat this process moving along the lashes to create a more pronounced curl.
- **Avoiding Damage**: Be gentle when using the curler to avoid pulling out or breaking your lashes. Curling after mascara application can lead to lashes sticking to the curler and being pulled out.

Choosing Mascara

- **Type Based on Desired Effect**:
    - **Lengthening Mascara**: Ideal for short lashes, these mascaras have dense bristles that allow you to get closer to the roots for an elongating effect.
    - **Volumizing Mascara**: These mascaras are perfect for thin lashes. They contain waxes and silicones that coat lashes, making them appear thicker and fuller.
    - **Curling Mascara**: If your lashes are straight, curling mascaras can help provide a lift and curve.
- **Waterproof Formulas**: Waterproof mascara is excellent for long-lasting wear and is resistant to smudging, which is ideal for humid conditions or emotional events. However, they require a good makeup remover to avoid tugging on your lashes during removal.

Application

- **Technique for Volume and Length**: Wiggle the mascara wand at the base of your lashes and then pull it through to the tips in a smooth motion. This technique coats every lash and adds both length and volume.
- **Building Intensity**: For a more dramatic look, apply a second coat of mascara. Do this while the first coat is still wet to avoid clumping.
- **Preventing Clumps**: If you notice clumps, use a clean spoolie or an eyelash comb to gently separate and define your lashes.

Lower Lashes

- **Subtle Definition**: Applying mascara to your lower lashes can define your eyes and balance the overall look. Use the tip of the mascara wand or a smaller brush for precision.
- **Light Application**: Be cautious with the amount of product on the wand to avoid clumps and smudging under the eyes. Consider using a waterproof formula for the lower lashes to prevent smudging throughout the day.

Additional Tips

- **Avoid Pumping the Wand**: Pumping the mascara wand in and out of the tube can dry out the mascara faster by introducing air into the tube.
- **Regular Replacement**: Replace your mascara every three to six months to prevent eye infections and ensure the best performance.
- **Customizing with Multiple Formulas**: Don't hesitate to layer different types of mascaras. For instance, you can use a lengthening mascara followed by a volumizing one for a customized effect.

Mascara plays a transformative role in eye makeup, significantly enhancing the appearance of your eyes. The key to achieving beautifully full lashes lies in choosing the right type of mascara, mastering the application technique, and properly preparing your lashes. This not only enhances your overall makeup look but also accentuates the natural beauty of your eyes. Remember, perfecting your mascara application is a matter of practice. Experiment with different formulas and techniques to find what best suits your style and lash type.

Eye makeup, with its endless creative possibilities, is an exciting realm to delve into. Whether your goal is a subtle enhancement or a striking, bold statement, the journey begins with mastering basic techniques. As you grow more confident in your skills, don't hesitate to experiment with new styles and colors. Each step in learning and experimenting brings you closer to achieving eye makeup looks that resonate with your personal aesthetic and enhance your natural beauty.

Chapter 9: Brow Shaping and Filling

Eyebrows play a crucial role in framing your face and enhancing your overall makeup look. Well-groomed and properly shaped brows can uplift your appearance, adding structure and balance to your facial features. In this chapter, we delve into the art of brow shaping and filling, guiding you through finding your perfect brow shape, selecting the right tools for grooming, and techniques for filling and defining your brows.

Finding Your Perfect Brow Shape

The quest for the perfect eyebrow shape is unique to each individual, as it significantly depends on your facial structure and natural brow line. Crafting the right brow shape can enhance your overall facial features, bringing harmony and balance to your appearance. Here's a more detailed approach to finding your perfect brow shape.

Understanding Face Shape

- **Tailoring to Your Face**: The shape of your face plays a pivotal role in determining the most flattering eyebrow shape. Each face shape has specific characteristics that can be accentuated or balanced with the right brow shape.
    - **Round Face**: If you have a round face, creating an angular brow with a higher arch can add definition and lengthen your face.
    - **Square Face**: For a square face, where the jawline is more pronounced, soft and rounded brows can create a gentle balance.
    - **Oval Face**: Oval faces often suit a variety of brow shapes, but a soft, natural arch works particularly well.
    - **Heart-Shaped Face**: Slightly rounded brows can complement a heart-shaped face by softening the pointed chin.
    - **Long Face**: For a longer face, extended horizontal brows can help to visually shorten the face.

Natural Brow Line as a Guide

- **Working with What You Have**: The natural shape and direction of your brow hairs are a great guide for shaping your brows. Observe the way your brows naturally grow and their starting and ending points.
- **Avoiding Over-Plucking**: It's important to avoid drastically altering your natural brow shape, as this can lead to an artificial look and potential over-plucking. Minor adjustments and clean-ups are usually sufficient.

Marking Key Points

- **Identifying Brow Landmarks**: Use a pencil or a makeup brush as a guide to mark the key points of your brows.
    - **Start of the Brow**: Align it vertically with the side of your nose. This is where your brow should ideally start.

- - **Brow Arch**: To find the natural arch, hold the pencil diagonally from the edge of your nostril, passing through the outer edge of the iris. This is typically the highest point of your brow.
  - **End of the Brow**: Continue the diagonal line from the nostril to the outer corner of your eye. This point marks the end of your eyebrow.
- **Symmetry Check**: Ensure both brows are as symmetrical as possible, but remember, minor differences are natural.

Consultation with a Professional

- **Expert Guidance**: If you're new to brow shaping or unsure about the best shape for your face, consulting a professional brow stylist can be incredibly beneficial. They can provide personalized advice and create a shape that complements your features.
- **Maintaining the Shape**: Once a professional has shaped your brows, you can maintain the look by plucking stray hairs that grow outside the defined shape.

Finding your ideal brow shape is a blend of art and science, taking into consideration your facial features and natural brow characteristics. By following these guidelines and perhaps seeking professional advice, you can define a brow shape that not only looks great but also feels authentically you. Remember, brows can make a profound impact on your overall look, so taking the time to shape them correctly is well worth the effort.

Tools for Brow Grooming

Well-groomed eyebrows can frame your face and enhance your overall appearance, making brow grooming an essential aspect of beauty care. To achieve and maintain perfectly shaped brows, it's important to have the right tools at your disposal. Here's a detailed exploration of the key tools you'll need for effective brow grooming.

Tweezers

- **Precision Removal**: A good pair of tweezers is indispensable for brow grooming. They are primarily used for plucking stray hairs that fall outside of your desired brow shape.
- **Slanted Tip Tweezers**: Look for tweezers with a slanted tip. This design offers a good balance between precision and ease of use, making them ideal for grasping and removing individual hairs.
- **Quality Matters**: Invest in a high-quality pair of tweezers with a firm grip and precise alignment to make plucking less painful and more efficient.
- **Regular Cleaning**: Remember to regularly clean your tweezers with alcohol to prevent bacterial buildup and ensure safe and hygienic grooming.

Brow Scissors

- **Trimming for Shape**: Small, sharp scissors are specifically designed for trimming eyebrows. They are useful for cutting longer hairs that may disrupt the overall shape and look of your brows.
- **Technique**: Comb your brow hairs upwards with a spoolie and then carefully trim only the tips of the hairs that extend beyond your desired brow shape. Be cautious not to over-trim, as it can create gaps or unevenness.

Spoolie Brush

- **Essential for Grooming and Shaping**: A spoolie brush resembles a clean mascara wand and is a crucial tool for brow grooming.
- **Blending Tool**: After applying brow products like pencils, powders, or gels, use a spoolie to blend the product into your brows. This helps create a more natural look by distributing the product evenly.
- **Identifying Uneven Areas**: Regularly brushing your brows can help identify areas that need trimming or filling. Brushing hairs upwards and outwards gives you a clear view of the natural brow shape and any sparse areas.

Brow Razors

- **Alternative to Plucking**: Brow razors are an excellent alternative for those who find tweezing too painful or have sensitive skin.
- **Precision Shaping**: They can be used for shaping the brows and removing fine hairs around the brow area with precision.
- **Gentle on Skin**: Unlike tweezers, razors can remove multiple hairs at once and are generally gentler on the skin. However, the results may not last as long as plucking.
- **Usage Caution**: When using a brow razor, hold the skin taut and use gentle, downward strokes. Be very careful to avoid nicks and cuts.

With these essential tools in your grooming kit, you can achieve well-maintained, beautifully shaped brows that enhance your facial features and elevate your makeup look. Each tool serves a specific purpose in the grooming process, from removing unwanted hairs to refining and shaping your brows. Remember, maintaining the condition of your tools and using them correctly is key to achieving the best results in your brow grooming routine.

Filling and Defining Brows

Creating perfectly defined and filled-in eyebrows is an essential skill in makeup artistry, as it frames the face and enhances your overall look. Here's a more comprehensive guide on how to fill and define your brows for a polished appearance.

Choosing the Right Product

- **Matching Color**: The first step in brow filling is choosing a product that closely matches your hair color and complements your skin tone. This ensures a natural and cohesive look.
- **Types of Brow Products**:
    - **Brow Pencils**: Great for precision and mimicking natural hair. Ideal for filling in sparse areas and defining the brow shape. Ensure the pencil is well-sharpened for fine, hair-like strokes.
    - **Brow Powders**: Provide a softer, more diffused look. Perfect for those who prefer a subtle enhancement or have naturally thick brows and just need to fill in a few areas.
    - **Brow Gels**: Useful for adding color and keeping brow hairs in place. Tinted gels offer color and hold, while clear gels are great for a more natural look.
    - **Brow Pomades**: Offer a more dramatic, defined look. They are excellent for sculpting and filling brows but require a bit more skill and a steady hand.

Filling Sparse Areas

- **Technique**: Use light, feathered strokes to fill in any sparse or thin areas in your brows. The goal is to mimic the natural growth of your brow hairs for a realistic appearance.
- **Building Up**: Start with less product and build up gradually. It's easier to add more product than to remove excess.

Defining the Shape

- **Outlining for Definition**: Lightly outline the edges of your brows to define the shape. Be careful not to make the lines too harsh; subtle definition is key.
- **Blending for Natural Finish**: After outlining, use a spoolie brush or a clean mascara wand to gently blend the product for a natural finish. Blending helps soften any harsh lines and evenly distributes the product.

Setting the Brows

- **Importance of Setting**: A brow gel is used to set the hairs in place and seal in the product. This step ensures your brows stay well-groomed and in shape throughout the day.

- **Application**: Apply the gel in short, upward strokes to coat the hairs evenly. For a more sculpted look, brush the hairs upwards and then smooth them out towards the tail of the brow.

Practicing Symmetry

- **Aiming for Balance**: While perfect symmetry isn't necessary (as natural brows are not exactly identical), aim for as much balance as possible between both brows.
- **Adjustments**: Make slight adjustments to each brow as needed to achieve a harmonious look. This may involve filling one brow more than the other or extending the tail of one brow slightly to match the other.

Mastering the art of brow shaping and filling is a transformative element in makeup application, significantly elevating your overall look. By understanding the right techniques and using suitable products, you can enhance your natural brow shape, effectively fill in sparse areas, and create a well-defined, polished appearance. This process of defining and filling brows can significantly uplift and accentuate your facial features, complementing both natural and dramatic makeup styles. It's important to remember that practice is crucial in mastering these skills. Over time, as you experiment with different tools and products, you'll develop an intuitive understanding of the amount of product needed and the techniques that best suit your unique brow shape and style. Patience and consistent practice are key to achieving perfectly polished and refined eyebrows, which can transform your makeup routine and enhance your natural beauty.

Chapter 10: Blush and Contouring Basics

Blush and contouring are essential techniques in makeup that enhance your facial structure and add a healthy glow to your complexion. This chapter focuses on how to select the right blush for your skin tone, introduces simple contouring techniques for beginners, and covers the basics of highlighting. These skills are fundamental in creating a balanced, dimensional, and vibrant makeup look.

Choosing Blush for Your Skin Tone

Selecting the perfect blush is an art that enhances your natural complexion and gives life to your makeup look. It's essential to consider both your skin's undertones and tone, as well as the formula that best suits your skin type. Here's a look at how to choose and apply blush to compliment your skin beautifully.

Understanding Skin Undertones

- **Importance of Undertones**: Knowing whether you have cool, warm, or neutral undertones is crucial in selecting a blush color that harmonizes with your natural skin color.
- **Matching with Undertones**: For cool undertones, which have hints of blue or pink, blushes in pink or rosy shades are ideal. They add a fresh pop of color that looks natural on your skin. Warm undertones, which lean yellow or golden, are beautifully complemented by peach or coral blushes, adding a warm, sun-kissed glow. Neutral undertones have the flexibility to experiment with both cool and warm spectrum blushes.

Considering Skin Tone

- **Adjusting to Skin Tone**: The intensity of the blush color should align with your skin tone. Lighter skin tones look best with softer shades, such as pale pink, light coral, or peach, as these shades provide a subtle, natural flush. Deeper skin tones can carry richer and more pigmented colors like deep coral, berry, or even a rich bronze, offering a stunning color payoff and enhancing the skin's natural warmth.

Blush Formulas

- **Types of Blushes**: Blushes come in powder, cream, and gel forms, each serving different skin types and desired finishes.
    - **Powder Blushes**: Ideal for oily or combination skin types, powder blushes offer a matte finish and are great for a more traditional blush application.

- - **Cream and Gel Blushes**: Perfect for dry or mature skin, these formulas provide a dewy, natural look. They blend seamlessly into the skin, offering a more hydrated and youthful appearance.
  - **Layering for Longevity**: For lasting power, you can layer different formulas. Start with a cream blush for a natural glow and top it with a powder blush to set it in place.

Application Tips

- **Where to Apply**: Apply blush to the apples of your cheeks – the part that raises when you smile. This placement gives a youthful and healthy look to your face.
- **Blending Technique**: Use a blush brush for powders or your fingers for creams and gels. Blend the product towards your temples in a light sweeping motion for a natural gradient. Avoid applying too close to the nose or dragging it down, as this can make your face look drawn.
- **Building Intensity**: It's best to start with a light hand and gradually build up the color. Over-application can be difficult to correct. For a more sculpted look, apply the blush slightly above the apples and blend upwards.

In conclusion, the right blush can significantly enhance your makeup, adding a healthy radiance and dimension to your face. By considering your skin's undertones and tone, and choosing a formula that complements your skin type, you can achieve a beautiful, natural-looking flush. Remember, the key to a perfect blush application is blending well and building color gradually to achieve the desired intensity.

Simple Contouring Techniques for Beginners

Contouring is a makeup technique used to define and enhance the natural structure of your face. It can seem daunting at first, but with some basic knowledge and practice, beginners can effectively contour to accentuate their best features. Here's a look at how to get started with contouring.

Identifying Face Shape

- **Understanding Your Face Shape**: The first step in contouring is to identify your face shape – be it oval, round, square, heart, or diamond. Each shape has different characteristics and areas that can be highlighted or receded to create a balanced look.
- **Customizing Contouring to Your Face**: Contouring techniques should be tailored to your specific face shape. For example, contouring under the cheekbones can add definition to round faces, while softening the edges of a square face involves contouring the jawline and forehead.

Product Selection

- **Choosing the Right Shade**: Pick a contouring product that is about two shades darker than your natural skin tone. This creates a natural shadow effect without looking harsh.
- **Creams vs. Powders**: Cream-based contour products are great for dry skin or for those seeking a more natural, dewy finish. Powder contours are ideal for oily skin and provide more precision and a matte finish. Beginners might find powders easier to control and blend.

Basic Contouring Steps

- **Cheekbones**: To define your cheekbones, apply the contour shade in the hollows beneath them. You can find this area by sucking in your cheeks and making a 'fish face'.
- **Jawline**: Contouring along the jawline can help to define and slim the face. Apply the contour along the jaw, blending downwards to create a subtle shadow.
- **Forehead**: For those with a larger forehead, apply contour along the hairline to create the illusion of a smaller forehead. The amount of contouring depends on the size of the forehead.
- **Nose**: Optional contouring along the sides of the nose can help it appear slimmer and more defined. This step requires a light hand and precision.

Blending is Key

- **Smooth Blending**: The most important aspect of contouring is blending. Use a contour brush or a damp beauty sponge to blend the product into your skin. The goal is to avoid any harsh lines or visible edges.
- **Direction of Blending**: Always blend contour in an upward motion to lift the face. Harsh downward blending can make the face appear dragged down.
- **Layering and Intensity**: Start with a small amount of product and build up gradually. It's easier to add more product than to remove excess.

Contouring can be a game-changer in makeup by enhancing your facial features and giving more dimension to your face. For beginners, the key is to start simple and practice regularly. Remember, the aim of contouring is to create subtle shadows and highlights that complement your natural face structure. With patience and practice, you'll soon be able to contour like a pro, achieving a beautifully sculpted and balanced look.

Highlighting Basics

Highlighting is a makeup technique used to enhance certain features of the face by adding light and creating an illusion of radiance and lift. When done correctly, highlighting can give your face a more defined, youthful, and glowing appearance. Here's a deeper exploration into the art of highlighting.

Creating a Glow

- **Purpose of Highlighting**: The main goal of highlighting is to draw attention to specific areas of the face by reflecting light. This can help enhance your best features and give your skin a luminous quality.
- **Key Areas for Highlight**: Common areas to apply highlighter include the tops of the cheekbones, which helps lift the face; the bridge of the nose, to create the illusion of a straighter nose; and the cupid's bow, to give the lips a fuller appearance. Other areas might include the brow bone, the center of the forehead, and the chin.

Choosing a Highlighter

- **Types of Highlighters**:
    - **Powder Highlighters**: These are the most common and are great for a more subtle, buildable glow. They are easy to apply and work well for most skin types, particularly oily skin.
    - **Liquid and Cream Highlighters**: These provide a more intense sheen and can create a dewy look. They are ideal for dry or mature skin, as they blend smoothly and don't settle into fine lines.
- **Color Selection**: Choosing the right color is crucial. Champagne and pearl tones work well for lighter skin, golden hues are beautiful on medium skin, and bronze or gold shades suit darker skin beautifully. The right shade will blend seamlessly with your skin and enhance your natural complexion.

Application Technique

- **Using the Right Tools**: For powder highlighters, a fan brush or a fluffy brush is ideal as it allows for light, even application. For creams or liquids, your fingertips or a damp beauty sponge can provide a more controlled and blended application.
- **Light Touch**: The key to highlighter is using a light hand. You can always build up the product for more intensity. Start with a small amount and gently apply it to the high points of your face.
- **Blending for a Seamless Finish**: Blend the edges of the highlighter into your skin or the underlying makeup for a seamless finish. Avoid leaving any harsh lines or obvious patches of product.
- **Layering with Other Products**: When using powder highlighter, apply it after your powder blush and bronzer. For creams and liquids, apply before any powder products to prevent the textures from clashing.

Highlighting, blush, and contouring are essential elements in makeup that, when applied correctly, can dramatically transform your appearance. Highlighting is not just about adding shimmer to the face; it's a strategic art of placing light to emphasize your best features, giving your skin a healthy, radiant glow. With practice, you can master the application technique, determine the right amount of product, and choose the ideal type of highlighter to complement your unique face shape and skin tone. The most flattering highlights are those that appear as a natural part of your skin, emanating an inner glow.

Similarly, blush and contouring add dimension and color, enhancing the overall structure and vitality of your face. Although these techniques might initially seem daunting, with regular practice, they can become enjoyable and a vital part of your makeup routine. Experimenting with various shades and formulas allows you to discover what best suits your individual style and complexion. The key to success in both blush and contouring lies in skillful blending, ensuring a seamless and natural finish. Together, these techniques contribute to a well-rounded and polished makeup look, highlighting your natural beauty and facial features in the most flattering way.

Chapter 11: Lip Makeup

Lip makeup is a crucial aspect of any beauty routine, offering the power to completely transform your look. Whether you prefer a natural tint or a bold statement lip, understanding the basics of lip makeup can greatly enhance your overall appearance. In this chapter, we'll explore how to choose the right lip colors, share tips for applying lipstick and gloss, and discuss the importance of lip care.

How to Choose Lip Colors

The right lip color can not only enhance your makeup look but also boost your confidence. However, with an overwhelming array of shades available, choosing the perfect lip color can be a challenge. Understanding a few key aspects can make this process easier and more enjoyable.

Understanding Undertones

- **Role of Skin Undertones**: Your skin's undertone is a crucial factor in determining which lip colors will be most flattering on you. Undertones are generally categorized as cool, warm, or neutral.
    - **Cool Undertones**: If your skin has cool undertones, you might notice hints of blue or pink beneath the surface. Lip colors with blue or purple bases, like berry shades, soft mauves, or rosy pinks, complement cool undertones beautifully.
    - **Warm Undertones**: Warm undertones are characterized by yellow, peach, or golden hues in the skin. If you have warm undertones, look for

lipsticks with orange or red bases, such as coral, warm pinks, or brick reds.
- **Neutral Undertones**: Those with neutral undertones have the most versatility, as they can pull off a wide range of colors. From nudes to reds to pinks, almost every color can look harmonious.

Considering the Occasion

- **Daytime vs. Evening**: The setting and time of day can influence your lip color choice. For daytime, especially in professional environments, subtle shades like nudes, light pinks, or peach tones are typically more appropriate. For evenings or special events, you can experiment with bolder shades like deep reds, plums, or even unconventional colors like bold purples or blacks for dramatic effect.

Complementing Your Makeup

- **Balancing Your Look**: Your lip color should harmonize with the rest of your makeup. If you're wearing heavy or dramatic eye makeup, a more subdued lip color can create a balanced look. Conversely, if your eye makeup is minimal, a bold lip can add a pop of color and focus to your look.

Seasonal Choices

- **Adapting to Seasons**: Just as your wardrobe changes with the seasons, so can your lip color preferences. Spring and summer tend to favor lighter, brighter shades, reflecting the playful and vibrant nature of these seasons. Think corals, bright pinks, or sheer glosses. During fall and winter, richer and deeper shades come into play, like burgundies, deep reds, and rich browns, mirroring the mood and colors of the colder months.

In conclusion, selecting the right lip color involves a blend of understanding your skin's undertones, considering the occasion, complementing your overall makeup, and being mindful of seasonal trends. Don't be afraid to experiment with different shades and finishes (matte, satin, gloss) to discover what looks best on you and reflects your personal style. The right lip color not only enhances your makeup but also helps to express your mood and personality.

Application Tips for Lipstick and Gloss

Applying lipstick and gloss correctly can enhance the overall look of your makeup, drawing attention to your lips and perfecting your smile. Here's a detailed guide on how to prepare your lips for application, and tips for applying both lipstick and lip gloss for a flawless finish.

Preparation

- **Importance of Prepping Lips**: Just like priming a canvas before painting, prepping your lips ensures a smoother application of lipstick or gloss. Well-prepared lips can significantly improve the appearance and longevity of your lip makeup.
- **Exfoliation**: Start by gently exfoliating your lips to remove any dead skin cells. You can use a lip scrub or a soft toothbrush to do this. Exfoliation helps in achieving a more even application and prevents the product from clinging to dry patches.
- **Moisturization**: Apply a hydrating lip balm after exfoliating. This step is crucial for keeping your lips moisturized, especially if you plan to use matte or long-wear lipsticks that can be drying. Allow the balm to absorb for a few minutes before applying lipstick.

Using Lip Liner

- **Defining Lips**: Lip liner is an essential step for achieving defined, polished lips. It creates a border that helps prevent color from bleeding and enhances the shape of your lips.
- **Matching Lip Liner**: Choose a lip liner that closely matches the color of your lipstick or a shade that matches your natural lip color. Outlining with a liner also provides a guide when applying lipstick and can help make the lips appear fuller or correct asymmetry.
- **Filling in Lips**: For added longevity and intensity, fill in your entire lips with the liner before applying lipstick. This creates a base that helps the color stay put longer.

Applying Lipstick

- **Method of Application**: Apply lipstick starting from the center of your upper lip, moving towards the edges, and then to the bottom lip. This ensures an even distribution of color.
- **Using a Lip Brush**: For more precision, especially with bold or dark shades, use a lip brush. A brush allows for more control and accuracy, especially around the lip edges and corners.
- **Blotting and Reapplication**: After the first application, gently blot your lips with a tissue and then apply a second layer. This technique helps in setting the first layer and makes the color last longer.

Applying Lip Gloss

- **Enhancing with Gloss**: Lip gloss can be used to add shine and a plump effect to your lips. Start by applying the gloss at the center of your lips and then spread it towards the outer corners.

- **Layering Over Lipstick**: Gloss can be applied over lipstick for added dimension and shine. Be careful not to blend the lipstick and gloss too much to maintain the color's integrity.
- **Natural Look**: For a subtle, natural look, wear gloss on its own. It gives a fresh and simple appearance, perfect for casual or minimal makeup days.

In summary, the key to perfect lip makeup lies in proper preparation, precise application, and understanding how to use products like lip liners, lipsticks, and glosses effectively. Each step, from exfoliating and moisturizing to outlining and filling, plays a crucial role in achieving beautiful, long-lasting lip color. With these techniques, you can experiment with different lip looks, from bold and dramatic to soft and natural, enhancing your overall makeup and showcasing your personal style.

Caring for Your Lips

Proper lip care is essential for maintaining soft, healthy lips and is the foundation for any successful lip makeup application. Your lips, unlike other parts of your skin, lack oil glands and are therefore more prone to drying out. Regular care and maintenance can prevent common issues like chapping, cracking, and dehydration. Here's a comprehensive approach to lip care, ensuring your lips remain in optimal condition.

Regular Exfoliation

- **Purpose of Exfoliation**: Regular exfoliation is key to removing dead skin cells from your lips, keeping them smooth and preventing flakiness. Smooth lips provide a better base for lipstick and gloss application.
- **Exfoliation Techniques**: Use a gentle lip scrub, which can be store-bought or homemade (using ingredients like sugar and honey). Alternatively, a soft toothbrush can be used to lightly brush over the lips. Be gentle to avoid irritation.

Hydration

- **Importance of Hydration**: Keeping your lips hydrated is crucial for their overall health. Hydration prevents cracking and peeling, ensuring your lips look plump and healthy.
- **Drinking Water**: Internal hydration is as important as external. Ensure you drink plenty of water throughout the day.
- **Using Lip Balms and Treatments**: Apply hydrating lip balms or treatments regularly. Look for ingredients like shea butter, vitamin E, and natural oils. During the day, opt for products with SPF to protect your lips from harmful UV rays.

Nighttime Care

- **Overnight Treatments**: Your skin, including your lips, goes into repair mode while you sleep. Applying a nourishing lip balm or treatment before bed can help repair and rejuvenate your lips overnight.
- **Richer Formulas**: Nighttime is a good opportunity to use thicker, more emollient lip care products that might be too heavy for daytime wear.

Avoiding Bad Habits

- **Preventing Dryness**: Habits like licking or biting your lips can strip them of moisture, leading to dryness and chapping. Saliva evaporates quickly, leaving lips drier than before.
- **Awareness and Alternatives**: Be conscious of these habits and actively try to stop them. Carry a lip balm with you to apply whenever you feel the urge to lick or bite your lips.

Lip Makeup and Care

- **Foundation for Lip Makeup**: Healthy, well-cared-for lips are the best canvas for any lip makeup, whether you're aiming for a natural look or a bold statement. Proper lip care enhances the effectiveness of lip makeup and contributes to a more polished overall look.
- **Incorporating Care into Routine**: Make lip care a regular part of your beauty routine, just like skincare. Consistent care not only improves the appearance of your lips but also enhances the application and wear of your lip makeup.

In conclusion, caring for your lips is a crucial aspect of your overall beauty regimen. By regularly exfoliating, hydrating, applying overnight treatments, and avoiding damaging habits, you can maintain the health and beauty of your lips. This, in turn, ensures that any lip makeup you apply looks its best, enhancing your facial features and complementing your overall makeup look. Remember, the effort you put into caring for your lips is just as important as the makeup you choose to apply on them.

Chapter 12: Everyday Makeup Looks

Navigating the world of makeup doesn't have to be complicated, especially when it comes to your everyday look. Whether you're heading to school, looking for a natural appearance, or preparing for a special occasion, there are simple yet effective makeup styles to suit your needs. In this chapter, we explore versatile everyday makeup looks that are easy to achieve and can be adapted to various settings and events.

School-Friendly Makeup

Creating a school-friendly makeup look is all about simplicity and subtlety. The goal is to enhance your natural beauty in a way that's appropriate for an academic setting and quick for those busy school mornings. Here's a detailed approach to achieving a fresh, understated look that's perfect for school.

Subtle and Simple

- **Philosophy**: School-friendly makeup focuses on accentuating your features subtly. It's not about bold transformations or dramatic statements but rather about looking effortlessly polished and natural.
- **Quick and Easy Application**: Choose products and techniques that are straightforward and time-efficient, making your morning routine as seamless as possible.

Basic Steps

1. **Skin**:
    - **Lightweight Coverage**: Opt for a tinted moisturizer or a BB cream instead of a full-coverage foundation. These products provide a natural, breathable coverage, evening out your skin tone without the heaviness of regular foundations.
    - **Concealer**: Use a lightweight concealer for areas that need a bit more coverage, like under-eye circles or blemishes. The key is to apply it sparingly and blend well so that it looks natural.
2. **Eyes**:
    - **Neutral Eyeshadow**: A light sweep of neutral eyeshadow can brighten your eyes without looking overdone. Choose shades that are close to your skin tone or slightly enhance it.
    - **Mascara**: A single coat of mascara can open up your eyes, making you look more awake. Opt for a non-clumping, lengthening formula.
    - **Eyeliner (Optional)**: If you choose to use eyeliner, a thin line along the lash line can define your eyes subtly. Stick to brown or grey liners for a softer look compared to black.
3. **Cheeks**:

- **Natural Blush**: A light application of blush can give you a healthy, youthful glow. Cream blushes are great for a dewy, natural look, while powders work well for a more matte finish. Smile and apply to the apples of your cheeks, blending towards the temples.
4. **Lips**:
   - **Tinted Lip Balm or Gloss**: Finish your look with a swipe of tinted lip balm or gloss. These products add a hint of color while keeping your lips hydrated. Choose shades that are close to your natural lip color for a subtle enhancement.

Less is More

- **Minimalist Approach**: The 'less is more' philosophy is key in school-friendly makeup. It's about using the least amount of product to achieve a noticeable yet understated effect.
- **Natural Enhancement**: Focus on products and colors that naturally enhance your features without drawing too much attention.

In summary, school-friendly makeup should be quick, easy, and natural-looking. It's about feeling confident and comfortable in your skin, with a minimal yet effective makeup routine. Remember, the best makeup is the kind that makes you feel like the best version of yourself, especially in a learning environment where comfort and simplicity are key.

Natural Look Tutorial

The natural makeup look, often described as 'effortlessly chic,' is a timeless style that suits any occasion. It emphasizes subtly enhancing your features, creating a look that's polished yet seemingly effortless. This style is perfect for those who want to look put-together without appearing as though they are wearing too much makeup. Here's a step-by-step guide to achieving a beautiful, natural makeup look.

Effortlessly Chic

- **Philosophy of Natural Makeup**: The essence of a natural makeup look is to accentuate your features gently without overpowering them. The aim is to look like a more refined version of your natural self.
- **Versatility**: This look is versatile, suitable for everyday wear, professional settings, and even special occasions where you want a subtle yet polished appearance.

Steps to Achieve the Look

1. **Base**:

-
    - **Light Foundation or Tinted Moisturizer**: Start with a light foundation or tinted moisturizer to even out your skin tone while keeping the coverage minimal. These products are ideal for creating a fresh, breathable base.
    - **Concealer**: Apply concealer sparingly and only in areas that need extra coverage, such as under the eyes, around the nose, or on blemishes. The goal is to cover imperfections subtly without masking your skin's natural texture.
2. **Eyes**:
    - **Matte Eyeshadows**: Choose matte eyeshadows in shades that are close to your natural skin tone. Subtle beiges, soft browns, or muted roses can add a bit of depth to your eyes without being too noticeable.
    - **Mascara**: Apply a light coat of mascara to enhance your lashes while keeping them natural-looking. Avoid volumizing or lengthening formulas that can look too dramatic for this look.
3. **Cheeks**:
    - **Cream Blush for Natural Flush**: Cream blushes blend into the skin for a more natural flush. Choose a color that resembles the natural color of your cheeks after a light exercise – often a soft pink, peach, or rose.
    - **Blending is Key**: Blend the blush well into the apples of your cheeks, ensuring there are no harsh lines or patches.
4. **Lips**:
    - **Nude or Pink Lipstick**: Select a lipstick in a nude or pink shade that closely matches your natural lip color. This enhances your lips without making them a focal point.
    - **Lip Balm Alternative**: For an even more natural look, opt for a tinted lip balm that provides a hint of color along with hydration.
5. **Finishing Touches**:
    - **Subtle Highlighter**: Apply a small amount of highlighter to the high points of your face – cheekbones and brow bones. This creates a subtle, healthy glow.
    - **Avoiding Over-Powdering**: If you need to set your makeup, use a light dusting of translucent powder on the T-zone. Avoid applying too much powder, which can make the skin look dry and less natural.

In conclusion, the natural makeup look is all about subtlety and enhancement. It requires a light hand and the right choice of products. This look is not about hiding your imperfections but rather about highlighting your natural beauty. Remember, the key to mastering this look is practice and understanding what works best for your unique features and skin type. With this approach, you can achieve an effortlessly chic appearance that's perfect for any day.

Makeup for Special Occasions

When it comes to special occasions, your makeup is an extension of your celebration. It's an opportunity to step out of your everyday makeup routine and indulge in a bit more glamour and elegance. Whether it's a wedding, a formal party, or an elegant dinner, special occasion makeup allows you to experiment with bolder colors and more dramatic techniques. Here's a step-by-step guide to creating a stunning makeup look for any special event.

Elevated Elegance

- **Enhanced Glamour**: Special occasions are perfect for experimenting with looks that may be too bold for your day-to-day life. This could mean more vibrant colors, higher levels of shimmer, or more dramatic contouring and highlighting.
- **Complementing Your Outfit**: Consider your outfit and the event's theme when planning your makeup. Your makeup should complement, not compete with, your overall look.

Creating the Look

1. **Foundation**:
   - **Long-Wearing Formula**: Choose a foundation that provides flawless coverage and has long-wearing capabilities. You want your base to remain intact throughout the event without needing frequent touch-ups.
   - **Preparation**: Ensure proper skin preparation before applying foundation. Use a primer suited to your skin type to create a smooth canvas and help your foundation last longer.
2. **Eyes**:
   - **Eye Makeup Styles**: The eyes are often the focal point for special occasion makeup. Options include a classic smoky eye, sophisticated winged eyeliner, or glamorous shimmering eyeshadows.
   - **False Lashes**: False lashes can dramatically enhance your look, adding volume and length to your lashes. Choose a style that complements the shape of your eyes and the intensity of your eye makeup.
   - **Balance**: If you're going bold on the eyes, keep your lip color more subdued, and vice versa.
3. **Contour and Highlight**:
   - **Defining Features**: Use contouring to define your cheekbones, jawline, and the sides of your nose. Contouring can add depth and dimension to your face.
   - **Adding Radiance**: Apply highlighter to the high points of your face, like the tops of your cheekbones, the bridge of your nose, and the cupid's bow, to create a radiant glow.
4. **Lips**:
   - **Statement Lipstick**: Choose a lipstick that makes a statement. Bold reds, deep berries, or vibrant pinks can be stunning choices for special

occasions. Make sure to line your lips first to prevent the color from bleeding.
   - **Long-Lasting Formula**: Opt for a long-lasting lipstick formula to minimize the need for reapplication.
5. **Setting the Makeup**:
   - **Locking in the Look**: Use a good quality setting spray to lock your makeup in place. This helps to ensure your makeup stays flawless throughout the event.

Confidence and Personal Style

- **Embracing Your Style**: The most important aspect of special occasion makeup is to wear it with confidence. Whether you choose a bold or a subtle look, it should reflect your personal style and make you feel comfortable.
- **Practice Makes Perfect**: If you're trying a new technique or color, practice the look a few times before the actual event to ensure you are comfortable and happy with the outcome.

Special occasion makeup is all about celebrating yourself and the event you're attending. It's a time to experiment, have fun, and let your personality shine through your makeup choices. Remember, the key to a successful look is not just in the products you choose, but in how they make you feel. With the right approach, you can create a look that is both glamorous and true to your individual style.

Chapter 13: Mastering Diverse Makeup Styles - Tutorials for Every Look

Quick and Easy Everyday Makeup Routine

1. **Primer**: Start with a primer for longer-lasting makeup. Apply it around the nose, chin, and forehead. Choose a primer that offers a radiant glow.
2. **Foundation**: Opt for an affordable, everyday foundation. Apply with a sponge for quicker and smoother coverage.
3. **Concealer**: Use a concealer for blemish coverage and under-eye dark circles. Apply gently and blend with a sponge.
4. **Powder**: Set the makeup with a translucent powder, focusing on oily areas and over the concealer. Skip baking to save time.
5. **Eyebrows**: Fill in sparse areas of the eyebrows to frame the face. Use a product that's quick and easy to apply.
6. **Mascara**: Choose a volumizing mascara to make the eyes look more awake.
7. **Bronzer**: Apply a light bronzer to add warmth and dimension. Use a fluffy brush for application on the cheekbones and forehead, opting for a lighter shade for natural results.
8. **Highlight**: Use highlighter with the same brush used for powder. Apply to areas like the cheekbones and brow bone for a subtle glow.
9. **Lips**: Opt for a moisturizing lip product for hydration and a slight shine. This step can be easily done while on the move.
10. **Hair**: For quick styling, choose a top knot or use dry shampoo for added volume and freshness.

Additional Tips:

- Skip the blush if you're in a rush.
- The routine is designed for efficiency, not perfection.
- Remember to blend the foundation into the neck for a seamless look.
- A simple routine can still result in a polished appearance.

E-girl Makeup Tutorial

1. Start with a Cleansed Face:
- Begin with a clean face.
- Apply a facial primer to create a barrier between your skin and makeup.

2. Color Correcting and Foundation:
- Use a color-correcting moisturizer to reduce redness.
- Apply a full-coverage concealer for dark circles and blemishes.

- Use a foundation, and blend it with a makeup sponge.

3. Eyebrows and Bronzing:
- Fill in the eyebrows with a brow pomade. Shave the ends if preferred.
- Apply a bronzer for contouring.

4. Blush and Setting with Powder:
- Use a jelly-textured blush on the cheeks and blend.
- Set the makeup with a loose setting powder, focusing on the under-eye area, T-zone, and other oily parts.

5. Lipstick as Multi-Use Product:
- Apply red lipstick on the lips and cheeks for added color.

6. Eye Makeup:
- Use an eyeshadow palette. Blend red and pink shades into the crease for depth.
- Highlight the eyelids with lighter colors from the palette.
- Apply mascara to enhance eyelashes.

7. Eyeliner Techniques:
- Use a semi-dried eyeliner for initial application.
- Draw bold lines without hesitation for best results.
- Go over with a darker, long-lasting eyeliner for a sharper look.

8. Accentuating Eye Features:
- Use a white eyeliner pencil on the waterline and under the eyes.
- Draw faux eyelashes under the eye for emphasis.
- Apply blue eyeshadow under the eyes (optional for blue eyes).

9. False Eyelashes:
- Apply false eyelashes.

10. Highlighting and Nose Contouring:
- Apply a highlighter under the eyes, on the nose, eyebrows, and cheeks.
- Contour the nose for a "button nose" look.

11. Finishing Touches:
- Apply red lip gloss.
- Improvise with hair styling if necessary.

12. Completed Look:
Review the overall makeup and adjust as needed.

Step-by-Step "Sun-Kissed" Glowy Makeup Tutorial

Step 1: Skin Prep for a Sun-Kissed Glowy Makeup Look

Hydrating with a Serum

- **Choosing the Right Serum:** Opt for a hydrating serum that is lightweight yet effective. Look for key ingredients like niacinamide, known for its skin-smoothing and brightening properties, and hyaluronic acid, which is excellent for retaining moisture in the skin. These ingredients work together to create a hydrated, plump base for your makeup.
- **Application:** Start by cleansing your face to ensure it's free of any impurities or residue. With clean hands, apply a small amount of serum onto your fingertips. Gently pat the serum onto your face and neck, focusing on areas that tend to be drier. Allow the serum to fully absorb into your skin before moving to the next step. This not only hydrates your skin but also helps to create a smooth canvas for the rest of your makeup application.

Enhancing Glow with Nourishing Oil

- **Selecting an Oil:** After the serum, use a nourishing facial oil that complements your skin type. For a sun-kissed look, oils with a light consistency that don't leave a greasy residue are ideal. Ingredients like maracuja, argan, or jojoba oil are great options as they are known for their nourishing and skin-enhancing properties.
- **Application on Face, Chest, and Shoulders:** Take a few drops of the oil into your palms and rub them together to warm it up. Gently press and massage the oil onto your face, paying special attention to areas that need extra hydration. Extend the application to your neck, chest, and shoulders. This not only hydrates these areas but also adds a subtle, healthy glow, tying the look together and enhancing the sun-kissed effect. The goal is to achieve a radiant complexion that looks naturally luminous, not oily.

Tips for Effective Skin Prep:

- **Layering Products:** Always apply the thinnest, most fluid products first and build up to the thicker ones. This ensures each product is absorbed effectively without feeling heavy on the skin.
- **Allowing Time for Absorption:** Give each product a minute or two to sink in before applying the next. This prevents pilling and ensures maximum efficacy of each product.
- **Gentle Application:** Use gentle, upward strokes when applying products. This helps in boosting circulation and gives a natural lift to your skin.
- **Consistency is Key:** Regular use of these products as part of your daily skincare routine can improve your skin's overall health and appearance, making it look naturally radiant with or without makeup.

Step 2: Priming for a Sun-Kissed Glowy Makeup Look

Choosing and Applying a Primer

- **Selecting the Right Primer:** For a sun-kissed glowy makeup look, choose a primer that helps minimize pores and provides a smooth base for makeup. The primer should be lightweight and suitable for areas that tend to get oily or where makeup might settle into fine lines, like around the nose, chin, and forehead.
- **Application Technique:** After your skin is prepped with serum and oil, apply the primer. Focus on areas that need smoothing or where makeup longevity is crucial. Use a small amount and gently blend it into the skin using your fingertips or a makeup sponge. The primer should blend seamlessly without leaving any heavy or greasy feel.

Targeted Priming for Specific Concerns

- **T-Zone Attention:** If you have an oily T-zone, pay special attention to these areas while applying the primer. This helps in controlling shine throughout the day and keeps your makeup looking fresh.
- **Pore Minimization:** For areas with visible pores, like around the nose, gently press the primer into the skin to ensure it fills the pores, creating a smooth, even surface.

Additional Tips:

- **Less is More:** Avoid using too much primer, as it can make the skin feel heavy and affect how the makeup sits on your skin. A pea-sized amount is usually sufficient.
- **Allowing Primer to Set:** Give the primer a minute or two to set before proceeding with foundation or concealer. This helps in creating a lasting makeup look.
- **Skin Type Consideration:** Choose a primer formula that complements your skin type. For oily skin, look for mattifying primers, and for dry skin, hydrating primers work best.

Step 3: Foundation for a Sun-Kissed Glowy Makeup Look

Choosing and Applying a Lightweight Foundation or Concealer

- **Product Selection:** Opt for a radiant concealer or a lightweight foundation that offers a natural, skin-like finish. The key is to choose a product that enhances the skin's natural glow without masking it. Look for a shade that matches your skin tone for a seamless look.

- **Application Technique:** Apply the product sparingly, focusing on areas that need coverage, like the center T-zone, under the eyes, and around any blemishes or redness. Use a damp makeup sponge for blending, as it helps achieve a more natural, skin-like finish. The goal is to even out the skin tone while maintaining a luminous, fresh appearance.

Building Coverage

- **Layering for Coverage:** If you need more coverage in certain areas, build it up gradually with thin layers. Allow each layer to set before applying the next. This method prevents the makeup from looking cakey and maintains the glowy effect.
- **Blending Edges:** Ensure that the edges of the applied foundation or concealer are well-blended into the skin, especially around the jawline, hairline, and ears, for a natural transition.

Additional Tips:

- **Using Concealer for Contouring:** You can also use a slightly darker shade of the same product to add dimension to your face. Apply it to areas like the sides of the forehead, under the cheekbones, and along the jawline, then blend thoroughly.
- **Keeping It Light:** Remember, the essence of a sun-kissed look is light and natural, so avoid heavy application. The focus should be on enhancing your natural skin rather than covering it up.
- **Skin Type Consideration:** For oily skin, you might prefer a product with a semi-matte finish to control shine, while those with dry skin might opt for more hydrating formulas.

Step 4: Contouring and Bronzing for a Sun-Kissed Glowy Makeup Look

Selecting and Applying Contour and Bronzer

- **Product Selection:** For a natural, sun-kissed look, choose a bronzer or a darker shade of your foundation/concealer. The bronzer should be a few shades darker than your skin tone but still within a natural color range to mimic a natural sun-touched effect.
- **Application Technique for Contouring:** Use the darker shade to contour the perimeter of your face, focusing on areas like the sides of your forehead and below your cheekbones. This creates depth and dimension, enhancing the natural structure of your face. Blend well using a makeup sponge or a contour brush, ensuring there are no harsh lines.
- **Bronzing for a Sun-Kissed Effect:** Apply the bronzer to areas where the sun naturally hits your face, such as the top of your forehead, cheekbones, and jawline. Use a fluffy bronzing brush for a soft, diffused look. The goal is to warm up your complexion, giving it a healthy, sun-kissed glow.

Blending for a Natural Finish

- **Seamless Integration:** Ensure that the contour and bronzer are well-integrated into your foundation. Blend the edges thoroughly to avoid any stark lines or patches. The transition between your base and the bronzed areas should be seamless and natural-looking.
- **Layering for Intensity:** If you desire more intensity, build up the bronzer gradually with light layers. This approach allows for more control and maintains the overall natural and glowy aesthetic.

Additional Tips:

- **Contouring According to Face Shape:** Tailor your contouring technique to your face shape. For example, if you have a round face, contouring under the cheekbones can create a more defined look.
- **Bronzer as Eyeshadow:** For a cohesive look, you can lightly sweep the same bronzer across your eyelids. This ties the look together and enhances the sun-kissed effect.
- **Avoiding Over-Application:** Be mindful not to over-apply, as the aim is to achieve a natural, sunlit appearance. The contour and bronzer should enhance, not overpower, your natural features.

Step 5: Applying Blush for a Sun-Kissed Glowy Makeup Look

Choosing and Applying Blush

- **Product Selection:** Select a blush that complements a sun-kissed look, ideally in shades of rose or peach with a dewy finish. The blush should add a healthy color to the cheeks, contributing to the overall radiant glow.
- **Application Technique:** Smile to find the apples of your cheeks. Apply the blush to these areas, blending upwards towards the temples. This placement helps to lift the face and enhances the sun-kissed effect. Use a blush brush or fingers for a more natural, blended look. The blush should meld seamlessly with the bronzer, creating a harmonious, warm glow.

Building and Blending

- **Layering for Intensity:** If you prefer more color, build the blush gradually with light layers. This approach allows for control over the intensity and maintains the natural, glowy look.
- **Blending for a Seamless Finish:** Ensure that the edges of the blush are well-blended into the skin and with the bronzer. There should be no harsh lines or visible boundaries between the blush and the rest of your makeup.

Additional Tips:

- **Choosing the Right Shade:** Consider your skin tone when selecting a blush shade. Warmer, deeper shades work well for darker skin tones, while lighter, peachy tones are great for fairer skin.

- **Blush as Eyeshadow:** For a cohesive look, lightly sweep the same blush across your eyelids. This ties the look together and enhances the sun-kissed effect.
- **Avoiding Over-Application:** Be careful not to over-apply blush, as the goal is to achieve a natural, sun-flushed look. The blush should add to the radiance without dominating the makeup.

Step 6: Concealing for a Sun-Kissed Glowy Makeup Look

Selecting and Applying Concealer

- **Product Selection:** Choose a concealer that offers a radiant finish and is a shade or two lighter than your foundation. This will help brighten the under-eye area and highlight certain parts of your face.
- **Application Technique:** Apply the concealer in small amounts to areas that need extra coverage or brightening, such as under the eyes, around the nose, and on any blemishes. Use a damp makeup sponge or a concealer brush for blending. The key is to dab and blend gently to avoid disturbing the foundation underneath.

Highlighting with Concealer

- **Strategic Placement:** Besides concealing, use the product to highlight the high points of your face, like the bridge of the nose, the center of the forehead, and the chin. This adds dimension and enhances the sun-kissed effect.
- **Blending for a Natural Look:** Ensure that the concealer blends seamlessly into your foundation. There should be no visible lines or patches. The transition between the concealer and the foundation should be smooth and natural.

Additional Tips:

- **Layering for Coverage:** If you need more coverage, build it up gradually with thin layers, allowing each layer to set before applying the next. This prevents the makeup from looking heavy.
- **Setting the Concealer:** To prevent the concealer from creasing, you can lightly set it with a translucent setting powder. However, use a minimal amount to maintain the glowy look.
- **Choosing the Right Shade:** The concealer shade should complement your skin tone and foundation. It should be light enough to brighten but not so light that it looks unnatural.

Step 7: Setting for a Sun-Kissed Glowy Makeup Look

Choosing and Applying Setting Powder

- **Product Selection:** Opt for a translucent setting powder that provides a natural finish. The powder should be fine and lightweight to set the makeup without dulling the skin's natural glow.
- **Application Technique:** Use a large, fluffy brush to apply the powder. Focus on areas prone to oiliness or where makeup tends to crease, such as the under-eye area, T-zone (forehead, nose, and chin), and around the mouth. Apply with a light hand to avoid a cakey appearance.

Maintaining the Glow

- **Strategic Application:** To preserve the sun-kissed glow, avoid over-powdering. Only apply powder where absolutely necessary. The goal is to set the makeup for longevity while keeping the radiant finish of the skin.
- **Blending for a Seamless Finish:** Ensure that the powder blends seamlessly into your foundation and concealer. There should be no visible lines or patches. The transition between powdered and unpowdered areas should be smooth.

Additional Tips:

- **Using a Powder Puff for Touch-Ups:** For those who prefer not to use powder, a clean powder puff can be gently pressed onto areas that need shine control. This method helps absorb excess oil without adding more product.
- **Choosing the Right Powder:** If you have dry skin, look for hydrating powders or consider using powder sparingly. For oily skin, a mattifying powder can help control shine throughout the day.
- **Avoiding Powder on Highlighted Areas:** To maintain the luminosity, especially on the high points of the face (like cheekbones and brow bones), avoid applying powder on these areas.

Step 8: Highlighting for a Sun-Kissed Glowy Makeup Look

Selecting and Applying Highlighter

- **Product Selection:** Choose a liquid highlighter that complements the sun-kissed look. The highlighter should have a golden or peachy hue to enhance the natural glow of the skin.
- **Application Technique:** Apply the highlighter to the highest points of your face where the light naturally hits, such as the cheekbones, brow bones, bridge of the nose, and cupid's bow. Use a makeup sponge or your fingertips for application. Tap the product gently onto the skin to blend it seamlessly without disturbing the underlying makeup.

Enhancing the Glow

- **Layering for Intensity:** If you desire a more intense glow, build up the highlighter gradually with light layers. This approach allows for control over the luminosity and maintains the natural, sun-kissed look.
- **Blending for a Natural Finish:** Ensure that the highlighter blends smoothly into your skin and the rest of your makeup. There should be no harsh lines or visible patches. The transition between the highlighter and the foundation should be smooth and natural.

Additional Tips:

- **Choosing the Right Shade:** The highlighter shade should complement your skin tone. Warmer, deeper shades work well for darker skin tones, while lighter, pearlescent tones are great for fairer skin.
- **Avoiding Over-Application:** Be careful not to over-apply the highlighter, as the goal is to achieve a natural, radiant look. The highlighter should add to the glow without dominating the makeup.
- **Highlighter as Eyeshadow:** For a cohesive look, you can also apply a small amount of the same highlighter on your eyelids. This ties the look together and enhances the overall sun-kissed effect.

Step 9: Eye Makeup for a Sun-Kissed Glowy Makeup Look

Preparing the Eyelids

- **Base Application:** Use a small amount of a liquid or cream product (like a concealer) in a shade similar to your skin tone or slightly darker as an eyeshadow base. This helps to even out the eyelid color and provides a smooth canvas for the eyeshadow.
- **Setting the Base:** Lightly set the base with a neutral eyeshadow to prevent creasing and to extend the wear of your eye makeup.

Applying Eyeshadow

- **Natural Shades:** Choose eyeshadows in natural, warm tones like soft browns, golds, or peaches to complement the sun-kissed look. These shades should enhance the eyes subtly without overpowering.
- **Application Technique:** Apply a mid-tone shade on the eyelid and blend it into the crease. Use a lighter, shimmering shade on the center of the lid, brow bone, and inner corner of the eye to brighten and add dimension.

Defining the Eyes

- **Soft Eyeliner:** For a soft, defined look, mix two darker eyeshadow shades and apply them along the upper and lower lash lines using a flat brush. This technique offers a softer look than traditional eyeliner and maintains the overall natural appearance.

- **Mascara:** Apply a coat of mascara to the top lashes, focusing on the outer half to create a lifted, open-eye effect. Avoid using mascara on the bottom lashes to keep the look light and fresh.

Additional Tips:

- **Blending for a Seamless Look:** Ensure all eyeshadows are well-blended. Harsh lines or unblended patches can detract from the natural, sun-kissed effect.
- **Customizing to Eye Shape:** Adapt the eyeshadow placement to your eye shape. For example, if you have hooded eyes, concentrate the darker shades on the outer corners to create the illusion of depth.
- **Keeping It Balanced:** Remember, the focus is on creating a natural, sun-kissed look, so keep the eye makeup balanced and in harmony with the rest of your face.

Step 10: Brow Shaping for a Sun-Kissed Glowy Makeup Look

Selecting and Applying Brow Products

- **Product Selection:** Choose a brow pencil or a similar product that matches your brow color. If it has a dual side with a wax-based formula, it can help in shaping and setting the brows.
- **Application Technique:** Use the pencil side to lightly fill in any sparse areas and to define the shape of your brows. The goal is to enhance the natural shape of your brows rather than creating an overly dramatic look. If using a wax-based side, run it through your brows to coat the hairs lightly, then use a spoolie brush to shape and set them in place.

Creating a Natural Brow Look

- **Light, Feathered Strokes:** Apply the product with light, feathered strokes to mimic the natural hair of your brows. This technique helps in achieving a more natural, filled-in look.
- **Blending for Softness:** After applying the brow product, use a spoolie brush to blend and soften any harsh lines. This ensures that your brows look naturally full and well-groomed.

Additional Tips:

- **Tailoring to Your Brow Needs:** If you have naturally full brows, you may only need to use the wax side to shape and set them. For sparser brows, more filling in might be required.
- **Choosing the Right Shade:** The brow product shade should be close to your natural brow color. Going too dark can make the brows look harsh and out of place in a sun-kissed look.

- **Avoiding Over-Application:** Be careful not to over-apply the product. Overly filled or darkened brows can overpower the natural, glowy makeup style.

Step 11: Lip Makeup for a Sun-Kissed Glowy Makeup Look

Selecting and Applying Lip Products

- **Product Selection:** Choose a lip liner in a nude or natural shade that complements your skin tone. For the lipstick, opt for a color that matches the blush used on your cheeks, maintaining a cohesive sun-kissed theme.
- **Lip Liner Application:** Start by outlining your lips with the lip liner. This defines the shape of your lips and helps prevent the lipstick from bleeding. Fill in the lips lightly with the same liner to enhance the lipstick's staying power.

Applying Lipstick and Gloss

- **Lipstick Application:** Apply the lipstick, preferably in a creamy or satin finish, to add color to your lips. If using a blush as lipstick (as suggested in the tutorial), dab it onto the center of your lips and blend outwards for a natural, stained effect.
- **Adding Gloss:** For an added touch of radiance, apply a sheer gloss or a glossy lip oil. Focus on the center of your lips to create a fuller, plump look. The gloss should be non-sticky and lightweight to keep the lips comfortable.

Creating a Natural, Sun-Kissed Lip Look

- **Blending for a Soft Effect:** After applying the lip liner and lipstick, press your lips together and blend the edges with your fingertip for a soft, diffused look. This technique helps in achieving a more natural, sun-kissed effect.
- **Layering for Intensity:** If you desire more color intensity or shine, you can add more lipstick or gloss, building up gradually to your preference.

Additional Tips:

- **Harmonizing with Overall Makeup:** Ensure that your lip color harmonizes with the rest of your makeup, especially the blush and eyeshadow, to create a cohesive sun-kissed look.
- **Choosing the Right Shades:** Select shades that enhance your natural lip color and complement your skin tone. Warmer, peachy, or rosy shades typically work well for a sun-kissed look.
- **Maintaining Balance:** Keep the lip makeup balanced with the rest of your face. The focus should be on creating a harmonious, radiant look that embodies the essence of being sun-kissed.

Step 12: Final Touches for a Sun-Kissed Glowy Makeup Look

Assessing and Adjusting Makeup

- **Overall Assessment:** Take a moment to assess your makeup in good lighting. Look for areas that might need a bit more blending or additional color. The key is to achieve a balanced and harmonious look that embodies a natural, sun-kissed glow.
- **Adjusting as Needed:** If you find any areas that appear too shiny or oily, especially in the T-zone, gently press a clean powder puff onto these areas. This technique helps absorb excess oil without adding more product, maintaining the glowy look.

Enhancing Glow and Color

- **Reinforcing Blush or Bronzer:** If you feel that your face needs a bit more warmth or color, lightly reinforce the blush or bronzer. Use a light hand to maintain the natural, sun-kissed effect.
- **Highlighting High Points:** For an extra touch of radiance, you can add a bit more highlighter to the high points of your face, like the cheekbones or brow bones. This step enhances the glow and ties the whole look together.

Setting the Makeup

- **Optional Setting Spray:** If desired, use a setting spray to help your makeup last longer. Choose a spray that offers a dewy finish to enhance the sun-kissed look. Hold the bottle a few inches away from your face and mist lightly.

Additional Tips:

- **Harmony and Balance:** Ensure that all elements of your makeup work together harmoniously. The goal is to look effortlessly sun-kissed and radiant.
- **Natural Finish:** Avoid heavy or cakey makeup. The beauty of a sun-kissed look lies in its natural and fresh appearance.
- **Regular Check-ups:** Throughout the day, check your makeup and do quick touch-ups if necessary, especially if you have oily skin or are in a humid environment

Dewy Glass Skin Makeup Tutorial

Step 1: Skin Prep with Serum

1. **Choosing the Right Serum**: Select a hydrating serum that suits your skin type. Look for ingredients like hyaluronic acid for hydration or niacinamide for brightening.
2. **Application Technique**: Apply the serum evenly across your face, gently patting it in with your fingertips to encourage absorption.

Step 2: Radiance-Boosting Device

1. **Device Setup**: Turn on your radiance-boosting device and set it to a comfortable intensity level.
2. **Using the Device**: Gently move the device over your skin in circular motions. Focus on areas that need more radiance or hydration.

Step 3: Moisturizing

1. **Select a Moisturizer**: Choose a moisturizer that complements your skin type. For dry skin, look for richer creams; for oily skin, opt for lighter lotions.
2. **Application Method**: Apply the moisturizer in sections, ensuring each part of your face receives equal attention. This prevents over- or under-moisturizing different areas.

Step 4: Sunscreen Application

1. **Choosing Sunscreen**: Pick a broad-spectrum sunscreen with at least SPF 30.
2. **Proper Application**: Apply sunscreen generously, covering all exposed areas of the face and neck. Don't forget the ears and hairline.

Step 5: Foundation Application

1. **Foundation Choice**: Select a cushion foundation for a lightweight, natural finish. Match the shade to your skin tone.
2. **Application Tips**: Use a tapping motion with the cushion applicator for an even and smooth coverage. Blend well around the jawline and hairline.

Step 6: Setting with Powder

1. **Selecting Powder**: Choose a translucent setting powder to avoid a cakey look.
2. **Application Strategy**: Apply the powder with a fluffy brush, targeting areas prone to oiliness or creasing, like under the eyes and the T-zone. Use a light hand to maintain the dewy finish.

Step 7: Eye Makeup

1. **Reddish Eye Makeup**: Opt for a reddish eyeliner or eyeshadow to create a subtle, rubbed-eye effect.
2. **Eye Contouring**: Use a neutral or slightly darker shade to contour the eyes. Apply in the crease and along the lower lash line for depth.
3. **Adding Glitter and Shimmer**: Apply a small amount of glitter under the pupil for a sparkling effect. Use a shimmer liner along the lash line for added brightness.

Step 8: Lashes

1. **Curling and Mascara**: Curl your lashes for an uplifted look. Apply a waterproof mascara to avoid smudging and to hold the curl.
2. **Applying Individual Lashes**: Choose individual lashes for a natural look. Apply darker lashes on the outer corners and lighter ones towards the inner corners.

Step 9: Brows

1. **Brow Gel Application**: Brush your brows upwards and outwards with a tinted or clear brow gel. This creates a fuller, more natural look.
2. **Filling in Sparse Areas**: If needed, use a brow pencil to lightly fill in any sparse areas, mimicking the natural hair growth.

Step 10: Contour and Blush

1. **Cream Contour**: Use a cream contour product to define your facial features. Apply under the cheekbones, along the jawline, and at the temples.
2. **Cream Blush Application**: Choose a pink cream blush for a natural flush. Apply on the apples of the cheeks and blend towards the temples.

Step 11: Lips

1. **Lip Liner**: Outline your lips with a natural-colored lip liner. This defines the shape and prevents lipstick from bleeding.
2. **Lip Tint**: Apply a lip tint for a long-lasting color. Blot and reapply for more intensity.
3. **Lip Gloss**: Finish with a clear or light-colored lip gloss for a plump, glossy look.

Step 12: Final Touches

1. **Applying Face Gloss**: Use a clear face gloss on the high points of your face for an added glow.
2. **Setting Spray**: Mist your face with a hydrating setting spray to set the makeup and add an extra layer of moisture.

Step 13: Final Check

1. **Blending Check**: Ensure all makeup is well-blended, with no harsh lines or patches.
2. **Adjustments**: Make any necessary adjustments, like adding more blush or blending the eyeshadow.

Step 14: Enjoy Your Look!

1. **Final Look**: Admire your dewy, glass skin makeup in good lighting.

2. **Maintenance**: Carry blotting papers or a compact powder for touch-ups throughout the day if needed.

This tutorial provides a comprehensive guide to achieving a dewy, glass skin makeup look, emphasizing hydration, radiance, and natural beauty.

Glitter Eye Makeup Tutorial

Step 1: Prime Your Eyelids

- Begin by applying an eyelid primer to ensure your eyeshadow stays in place.

Step 2: Apply Eyeshadow Guards

- Place adhesive eyeshadow guards under your eyes to catch any fallout.

Step 3: Use a Light Base Color

- Start with a light, matte eyeshadow (like white) and apply it under the highest point of your eyebrow for a subtle highlight.

Step 4: Apply a Transition Color

- Choose a soft yellow or similar light eyeshadow as a transition color in your crease. This step is optional but recommended for a more blended look.

Step 5: Blend in a Pinky-Purple Shade

- Use a pinky-purple eyeshadow, blending it from the inner corner to the outer corner of your eyelid. This will be the main color for your crease.

Step 6: Apply a Sparkly Shade

- Choose a sparkly eyeshadow and apply it to your eyelid using your finger. Look for a shade with a beautiful blue sparkle for added effect.

Step 7: Add Glitter

- Press cosmetic glitter all over the eyelid with your finger. This will cover the underlying eyeshadow but add a glamorous sparkle.

Step 8: Remove Eyeshadow Guards

- Carefully remove the eyeshadow guards.

Step 9: Apply Gel Liner

- Draw a winged liner with a gel eyeliner. You can adjust the thickness and length according to your preference.

Step 10: Enhance the Liner

- Go over the gel liner with a matte liquid eyeliner to cover any glitter fallout.

Step 11: Lower Lash Line

- Apply a purple eyeshadow under your lower lash line with a flat definer brush. Blend it out with a small blending brush.

Step 12: Waterline

- Line your waterline with a pencil eyeliner in a shade that complements the purple eyeshadow.

Step 13: Apply Mascara

- Curl your lashes and apply your favorite mascara.

Step 14: Add False Lashes (Optional)

- For a more dramatic look, apply false eyelashes. This step is optional and based on your preference.

Final Step: Enjoy Your Look!

- Your glitter eye makeup is complete. Enjoy your sparkly, glamorous look!

Easy Everyday Eyeshadow Makeup Tutorial

Materials Needed:

- Eyeshadow quad (with two matte shades and two shimmer shades)
- One versatile eyeshadow brush (such as a blending brush)
- Eyeshadow primer
- Translucent powder
- Concealer brush
- Mascara

Steps:

1. **Prep Your Eyes:**

- Apply an eyeshadow primer across your eyelids, from the inner to the outer corners.
- Blend the primer with a concealer brush.
- Set the primer with a translucent powder, covering your entire eyelid and under-eye area.

2. **Apply Transition Shade:**
   - Use the lighter peachy shade from your eyeshadow quad.
   - Tap off excess powder from the brush before applying.
   - Blend the shade back and forth in the crease of your eyelid.
   - Build up the shade to your desired intensity.
3. **Define the Outer Lid and Lower Lash Line:**
   - Pick up more of the same peachy shade.
   - Pat it onto the outer part of your eyelid, blending into the crease.
   - Use the tip of the brush to apply the same shade along your entire lower lash line.
4. **Deepen the Outer Lid:**
   - Use a deeper brown shade from the quad.
   - Pat it onto the outer part of your lid to add depth.
   - Blend it into the outer crease with circular motions.
   - Apply a bit of this shade on the outer part of your lower lash line.
5. **Add Shimmer to the Lid:**
   - Clean your brush using a brush cleaner.
   - Pick up a peachy shimmer shade on the flat side of the brush.
   - Apply it to the inner part of your lid, starting with a packing motion and then blending.
6. **Highlight Inner Corner and Brow Bone:**
   - Use a light highlighter shade from the quad.
   - Apply it to brighten the inner corner of your eyes and just under your brow bone.
7. **Finish with Mascara:**
   - Curl your lashes if desired.
   - Apply your favorite mascara, focusing on grabbing each lash for a full effect.
8. **Final Touches:**
   - You can add eyeliner or keep it simple with just the eyeshadow and mascara.
   - Adjust the intensity of the shades according to your preference for a more natural or dramatic look.

Tips:

- For hooded eyes, ensure the transition shade is visible above the lid.
- Holding the brush towards the end gives a lighter application.
- Use a finger for more intense shimmer or a brush for a softer look.
- Practice blending to achieve a seamless transition between shades.

This tutorial should help you achieve a soft, everyday eyeshadow look perfect for any occasion!

Glossy Lips Makeup for Teens

1. **Preparation**: Start with clean, moisturized lips. Use a gentle lip scrub if necessary to remove any dead skin, and follow up with a hydrating lip balm.
2. **Base Application**: Apply a light layer of foundation or concealer over your lips. This helps to create an even base and can make your lip color last longer.
3. **Lining the Lips**: Choose a lip liner that closely matches your natural lip color or the gloss you'll be using. Carefully outline your lips to define their shape. You can slightly overline for a fuller look, but remember to keep it natural, especially for teens.
4. **Applying Lip Color**: Pick a lip color that complements your skin tone. For a more natural look, opt for nude or light pink shades. Apply the lipstick evenly on your lips, staying within the lines you've drawn.
5. **Adding Gloss**: Now for the glossy effect! Apply a clear or slightly tinted lip gloss over your lipstick. Start at the center of your lips and work your way outwards. Be careful not to apply too much gloss, as it can get sticky.
6. **Final Touches**: For a clean and polished look, use a small brush with a bit of concealer to clean up any edges or smudges around your lips.
7. **Hydration**: Throughout the day, keep your lips hydrated. If you feel the gloss wearing off, you can reapply a small amount, but make sure your lips don't dry out.

Remember, the key is to enhance your natural beauty and feel comfortable with your look. Experiment with different shades and amounts of gloss to find what works best for you!

Graphic Eyeliner Makeup Tutorial

Materials Needed:

- Black liquid eyeliner with a fine, pointy brush
- Black eyeshadow (optional)
- Smudging brush (optional, for smudging)
- False eyelashes (optional, for added effect)

Steps:

1. **Prepare Your Eyeliner**: Choose a black liquid eyeliner that has a fine, pointy brush for precise application.

2. **Line the Entire Lash Line**: Start by carefully lining your entire lash line. This step is important to create a seamless look, especially if you're planning to wear false eyelashes.
3. **Draw the Wing**: From the outer corner of your eye, extend a winged line. Make a flick outward and then connect it back to the lash line. This forms the base of your winged eyeliner.
4. **Create the Graphic Element**: Look straight ahead to find where your eyelid crease ends. Draw a line from this point to the end of the wing, using small, controlled strokes. This line adds the graphic effect to your eyeliner.
5. **Tightline Your Eyes**: (Optional) For added intensity, tightline your upper lash line.
6. **Smudge and Mattify**: (Optional) If you prefer a softer look, use a black eyeshadow with a smudging brush to gently soften and mattify the eyeliner.
7. **Apply False Eyelashes**: (Optional) For a dramatic effect, apply a pair of false eyelashes. Choose lashes that flare at the ends to enhance the winged effect.
8. **Finalize Your Look**: Check both eyes for symmetry and make any necessary touch-ups. Your graphic eyeliner look is now ready!

Tips:

- Practice is key to mastering this look. Don't be discouraged if it takes a few tries to get it right.
- Keep makeup remover and cotton swabs close by for quick corrections.
- Feel free to adjust the angle and length of the graphic line to suit your eye shape best

Eyeliner Tutorial for Beginners

Materials Needed:

- Eyeliner (preferably a liquid eyeliner pen for ease of use)
- A dual-sided mirror (with both magnifying and standard views)
- A small, flat surface (like a plastic lid) for preparing the eyeliner
- A small, fine-tipped brush (like a lip brush) and a cotton swab
- Gentle eye makeup remover (water-based recommended)
- Eyeshadow (optional, for corrections)

Step 1: Preparation

1. **Select the Right Mirror**: Use a dual-sided mirror to check your eyeliner application from different perspectives.

2. **Stabilize Your Hand**: Rest your elbow on a stable surface to keep your hand steady.
3. **Use Your Pinky for Additional Support**: Rest your pinky on your cheek or near your eye for better control.

Step 2: Practice Strokes

1. **Dry Run**: Practice making small strokes in the air near your lash line to get used to the motion.

Step 3: Prepare the Eyeliner

1. **Prime the Eyeliner Pen**: Press the tip of the eyeliner pen against a small, flat surface to ensure it is well-coated with the eyeliner liquid.

Step 4: Application

1. **Start in the Middle**: Begin by applying the eyeliner at the middle of your lash line.
2. **Extend Outward**: Draw the line outward from the center, keeping the eyeliner pen as parallel as possible to your lash line.
3. **Inner Corner Precision**: For the inner corner, keep the line very fine. Start where your lashes begin, avoiding the innermost corner.
4. **Ensure Smoothness**: Use your pinky for stability to maintain a smooth, steady line.

Step 5: Subtle Enhancement

1. **Adjust to Preference**: You can vary the thickness of the line according to your preference, aiming for a subtle look that defines your eyes.

Step 6: Correcting Mistakes

1. **Use a Fine-Tipped Brush and Cotton Swab**: If you make an error, use a fine-tipped brush with a bit of makeup remover to gently correct it.
2. **Clean Up**: Use a dry cotton swab to dab away any excess remover and prevent smudging.
3. **Touch-Up as Needed**: If the eyeliner leaves a stain, reapply your base eyeshadow or use a light-reflective eyeshadow to cover any imperfections.

Step 7: Finishing Touches

1. **Enhance with Mascara or False Eyelashes**: Complete your look with a coat of mascara or by applying false eyelashes for added impact.

Tips:

- Practice is key. Don't get discouraged if it doesn't turn out perfect on the first try.

- Keep your hand as steady as possible for a smoother application.
- This technique is about enhancing your natural eye shape and beauty.

Bold Eyebrow Tutorial

1. Brush Your Brows:

- Begin by brushing your eyebrows upwards using a brow spoolie. This step is crucial for defining the natural shape of your eyebrows.

2. Outline with Brow Pencil:

- Use a brow pencil to create a subtle outline.
- Draw a fine line just underneath the brow.
- Use the spoolie to blend the line, ensuring there are no harsh lines.
- Start filling in any sparse areas to make your brows appear fuller.
- Pay special attention to defining the shape, particularly the arch, to create the illusion of a more pronounced arch.

3. Apply Brow Pencil Sparingly:

- Apply the brow pencil lightly on the inner third of your brow. The majority of the product should be applied towards the outer part of the brow.

4. Use Eyebrow Gel for Definition:

- With an angled brush, apply eyebrow gel to add definition.
- Gradually build up the color and definition on the outer part of your brow.
- Use small, light strokes for an even application, focusing mainly on the outer half of the brow.

5. Apply Clear Brow Gel:

- Next, apply a clear brow gel.
- Brush the inner brow hairs upwards.
- For the rest of the brow, brush the hairs in their natural growth direction.

6. Define with Concealer:

- Apply a cream concealer just underneath the brow to enhance its definition and structure.
- Blend the concealer well for a smooth finish.
- Use any remaining concealer on the brush to tidy up and define the top of the brow, but be careful not to apply too much.

7. Final Look:

- Review your brows for any final adjustments.
- Aim for a smooth transition from light to dark, with a well-defined and structured appearance.

Conclusion:

- This bold brow style is perfect for a full makeup look and when you desire a more dramatic eyebrow appearance.

Everyday Eye Makeup Tutorial

Creating a beautiful everyday eye makeup look doesn't have to be complicated. Here's a simple, step-by-step guide to enhance your eyes quickly and effectively:

1. Start with an Eyeshadow Primer:

- Begin by applying an eyeshadow primer to your lids. This helps your eyeshadow stay put throughout the day and makes the colors pop.

2. Use Eyeshadow Guards:

- Place eyeshadow guards under your eyes. These handy tools catch any fallout from your eyeshadow application and help create a neat line for your eyeliner.

3. Apply a Neutral Base Eyeshadow:

- Choose a light, neutral eyeshadow shade for your base. Sweep it across your crease, blending from the inner to the outer corner. This step creates a warm, natural depth.

4. Add a Touch of Shimmer:

- For a bit of sparkle, apply a soft pink or similar shimmery shade to your eyelids. Using your finger can give you better control and more intense color payoff.

5. Define with Gel Eyeliner:

- With a gel eyeliner and an angled brush, draw a smooth line right above your upper lash line. If you're feeling confident, extend this line into a winged tip at the outer corner of your eye.

6. Deepen with Dark Eyeshadow:

- Using a small brush, smudge a dark brown eyeshadow above your eyeliner. This adds depth and a smoky effect to your lash line.

7. Clean Up with Concealer:

- Apply a small amount of concealer beneath your winged liner to sharpen and define the line. This step also helps clean up any smudges or fallout.

8. Waterline with Eye Pencil:

- Line your waterline with a copper or brown eye pencil. This step adds warmth to your eyes and makes them stand out.

9. Curl Lashes and Mascara:

- Curl your eyelashes for an open, awake look. Follow up with a coat of volumizing mascara to both your upper and lower lashes.

10. Optional: Apply False Lashes:

- For added drama, you can apply a pair of false lashes. Choose a style that complements your natural lash line and enhances your eye shape.

11. Final Adjustments:

- Take a moment to check your makeup in good lighting. Make any necessary touch-ups to ensure a seamless and polished look.

12. Ready to Go:

- Your everyday eye makeup is now complete! This look is versatile and suitable for various occasions, from a day at the office to an evening out.

Remember, makeup is a form of self-expression, so feel free to adapt these steps to suit your personal style and preferences. Enjoy experimenting!

Natural Glam Teenager Makeup Tutorial

1. Preparation

- **Eyebrow Shaping**: Shape the eyebrows to enhance the eye area. Professional shaping is recommended for best results.

2. Eye Makeup

- **Eyeshadow Primer**: Apply an eyeshadow primer to the eyelids.
- **Base Eyeshadow**: Use a neutral eyeshadow palette. Apply a base color all over the eyelid.
- **Crease Definition**: Choose a dusty mauve shade and apply it lightly into the crease.
- **Lid Color**: Opt for a lighter pink shade. For more intensity, dampen the brush with a setting spray before application.
- **Outer Lid**: Apply a darker eyeshadow to the outer half of the lid and blend into the outer V.
- **Eyeliner**: Use a dark eyeshadow with a slanted brush to line the lashline for a softer look.

3. Eyebrows and Lashes

- **Eyebrow Filling**: Fill in the eyebrows using an eyebrow pencil that matches your hair color.
- **Mascara**: Curl the lashes and apply mascara. For added effect, consider using false eyelashes.

4. Face Makeup

- **Foundation**: Apply a BB cream for light coverage.
- **Concealer**: Use a concealer under the eyes and blend with fingers for a natural finish.
- **Setting Powder**: Lightly set the face with a translucent powder.
- **Blush**: Apply a light blush to the cheeks.
- **Highlighter**: Use a highlighting palette on the tops of the cheeks, blending well.

5. Lips

- **Lipstick**: Choose a natural-looking lipstick.

6. Finishing Touches

- **Lower Lash Mascara**: Apply a bit of mascara to the lower lashes for a complete look.

Tips:

- This look is suitable for special occasions like dances or weddings.
- Focus on blending and enhancing natural beauty.

Teen Makeup Tutorial for Beginners

1. Preparation

- **Skin Care**: Start with a clean face. Apply a moisturizer suited for teenage skin. Even if you have oily skin or acne, use an oil-free moisturizer to keep your skin hydrated.

2. Foundation

- **Tinted Moisturizer**: Use a tinted moisturizer instead of a heavy foundation. Apply a small amount with a brush in circular motions, ensuring it blends well into the skin, especially around the hairline and jawline.

3. Concealer

- **Spot Concealing**: For covering blemishes, apply concealer with a finger or a sponge, dabbing gently on the spots. Avoid applying concealer directly from the container to the face to prevent the spread of bacteria.

4. Blush

- **Applying Blush**: Use a cream blush for a natural look. Apply a small amount with the same brush used for the tinted moisturizer for a well-blended finish.

5. Bronzer (Optional)

- **Application**: If desired, lightly apply bronzer with a big brush to areas where the sun naturally hits your face (forehead, nose, chin, and cheeks).

6. Highlighter (Optional)

- **Cream Highlight**: Apply a small amount of cream highlighter to the cheekbones and a little on the nose for a natural glow.

7. Eyeshadow

- **Natural Colors**: Choose natural colors like oranges, golds, and browns. Apply a base color all over the lid, then use a darker color on the outer third of the eye. Blend well to avoid harsh lines.

8. Eyebrows

- **Grooming**: Use a clear mascara to comb through the eyebrows. Brush upwards and then shape along the top of the brow line.

9. Lips

- **Lip Gloss**: Finish with a neutral-colored lip gloss. Apply within the natural lip line for a subtle shine.

10. Mascara (Optional)

- **Application**: Apply mascara sparingly, using a zigzag motion from the base to the tip of the lashes. Use a lash comb to remove clumps.

11. Eyeliner (Optional)

- **Soft Application**: For a subtle look, apply eyeliner to the outer section of the eye. Smudge gently with a finger for a softer effect.

12. Finishing Touches

- **Mistakes**: In case of any mascara smudges, wait for it to dry and then gently brush it off with a makeup brush.

13. Aftercare

- **Removing Makeup**: Always remove makeup at the end of the day. Follow up with a skin cleanser and moisturizer.

Tips:

- **Experiment at Home**: Feel free to experiment with different looks at home.
- **Natural Beauty**: Emphasize your natural features and avoid overdoing makeup.
- **Healthy Skin**: Keep your skin healthy by following a regular skincare routine.

As we wrap up this chapter, I hope you've found inspiration and confidence in exploring the diverse world of makeup. Whether you were drawn to the quick and easy everyday routines or the more detailed and dramatic E-girl looks, my goal has been to equip you with the knowledge and techniques to express your unique style.

We started with the essentials of everyday makeup, focusing on creating a polished look efficiently. The tips and tricks shared here are designed to streamline your routine, ensuring you look your best even when time is short. Remember, makeup doesn't always have to be about perfection; it's about enhancing your natural beauty and feeling great.

For those of you who love to experiment and make bold statements, the E-girl makeup tutorial offered a playground of vibrant colors and dramatic styles. It's all about self-expression and having fun with your look. Don't be afraid to step out of your comfort zone and try something new.

The "Sun-Kissed" and "Dewy Glass Skin" tutorials brought us into the realm of luminous and radiant skin. These looks are all about starting with a well-prepped skin base, highlighting the importance of skincare in makeup. Achieving that glow isn't just about the products you apply; it's about taking care of your skin from within.

And to our younger readers, the teenager-focused tutorials were crafted with your needs in mind. Makeup during these years should be about exploration, learning, and most importantly, enhancing your natural beauty. You're at a wonderful stage of life where you can play with trends and discover what works for you.

As we close this chapter, I encourage you to keep practicing and experimenting. Makeup is an ever-evolving art form, and you are your own best artist. Each style we've covered is more than just a set of steps; it's a way to showcase your personality and creativity. So embrace these diverse styles, enjoy your makeup journey, and let the world see the beauty that is uniquely yours.

Chapter 14: Advanced Techniques - Elevating Your Makeup Mastery

Welcome to Chapter 14, where we dive into the world of advanced makeup techniques. This chapter is designed for those of you who are ready to take your makeup skills to the next level. Whether you've been practicing for a while or simply have a passion for learning more intricate makeup methods, this is the perfect place for you. We're going to explore some of the most iconic and sought-after makeup styles, breaking them down into manageable steps. Let's embark on this exciting journey together, enhancing your artistry with each brushstroke.

Smokey Eye Tutorial

The smokey eye is a classic look that never goes out of style. It's versatile, glamorous, and perfect for making a statement. But, it can be a bit intimidating if you're not sure where to start. Fear not! I'll guide you through the process of creating a flawless smokey eye. We'll talk about choosing the right shades for your eye color, blending techniques, and how to prevent fallout. Remember, the key to a great smokey eye is blending – the smoother the gradient, the more polished the look.

Ah, the smokey eye – an iconic look that exudes glamour and sophistication. It's a favorite for red carpet events, nights out, and whenever you want to add a touch of drama to your look. If you've been hesitant to try it out, let's change that. I'm here to walk you through each step, ensuring you can achieve a stunning smokey eye that complements your eye color and personal style.

Step 1: Eye Color and Shade Selection

- **Complementary Shades**: The key to a beautiful smokey eye is choosing shades that complement your natural eye color. For brown eyes, rich plums or bronzes add warmth; for blue eyes, try warm browns or golds; and for green or hazel eyes, purples or deep greens work wonders.
- **Palette Selection**: Typically, you'll need three shades – a light highlight color, a medium base color, and a dark smokey color. Choose a palette where these shades seamlessly blend into each other.

Step 2: Priming Your Lids

- **Eye Primer**: Apply an eyeshadow primer over your lids. This step is crucial for ensuring your smokey eye stays put and doesn't crease or smudge.
- **Base Shadow**: Apply a neutral or light eyeshadow over the primer. This base helps with blending and intensifies the colors you'll apply next.

Step 3: Building the Base

- **Medium Shade Application**: Take the medium shade from your palette and apply it across your eyelid, up to the crease. Use a flat eyeshadow brush for this step for even coverage.

Step 4: Creating the Smokey Effect

- **Dark Shadow Application**: Now, it's time to get smoky. Using a smaller, more precise brush, apply the darkest shade to the outer corner of your eye and into the crease. Create a 'V' shape at the outer corner and blend inward.
- **Blending is Key**: The most crucial aspect of a smokey eye is blending. Use a clean blending brush to smooth out any harsh lines, particularly where the dark shade meets the medium shade. The goal is a gradient effect with no obvious borders between colors.

Step 5: Lower Lash Line

- **Smoking Out the Lower Lash Line**: Using the same dark shade, lightly smudge along your lower lash line with a small brush. This step balances the look and adds to the smoky allure.

Step 6: Highlighting

- **Inner Corner and Brow Bone**: Apply the lightest shade to your inner corners and just beneath your brows. This highlight creates contrast and makes the eyes pop.

Step 7: Eyeliner

- **Lining the Eyes**: For added drama, line your upper lash line with a black eyeliner. You can also line your waterline for a more intense look. Smudge the line slightly with a brush or a smudging tool for a softer edge.

Step 8: Mascara and Finishing Touches

- **Mascara Application**: Apply generous coats of volumizing mascara to both your upper and lower lashes. False lashes are optional but can elevate the look even further.
- **Clean Up**: If there's any fallout under your eyes, clean it up with a bit of concealer.

Additional Tips:

- **Practice Makes Perfect**: Don't be discouraged if it doesn't turn out perfect the first time. Practice is key to mastering the smokey eye.
- **Work in Light Layers**: Build the intensity gradually. It's easier to add more product than to remove excess.

- **Choose the Right Brushes**: Use different brushes for different steps – a flat brush for application, a smaller brush for precision, and a fluffy brush for blending.
- **Setting Spray**: To ensure longevity, you can spritz your brush with a setting spray before dipping into the shadow.

Creating a smokey eye is like painting – it's about blending colors and creating depth. Remember, makeup is a form of expression and artistry. Have fun with it, experiment with different colors and intensities, and most importantly, wear your smokey eye with confidence. You're about to own one of the most timeless looks in makeup history!

Contouring and Highlighting Like a Pro

Now, let's talk about sculpting your face. Contouring and highlighting are like the magic wands of makeup; when done correctly, they can enhance your natural beauty and facial structure in remarkable ways. But, as with any magic trick, they require skill, understanding, and a bit of practice. Let's delve into how you can master these techniques, tailored to your unique face shape and features.

Understanding Your Face Shape

- **Identifying Face Shape**: The first step is to determine your face shape – oval, round, square, heart, or diamond. Stand in front of a mirror with your hair pulled back and observe the widest parts of your face, the shape of your jaw, and the overall length of your face.
- **Customizing Techniques**: Each face shape has different contouring and highlighting needs. For example, round faces benefit from contouring along the sides of the forehead and jawline to create more defined angles, while heart-shaped faces may require contouring near the chin to balance out the forehead.

Selecting Products

- **Types of Products**: You have a variety of options – creams, powders, and sticks. Creams are great for dry skin and create a dewy finish; powders are ideal for oily skin and provide a matte finish; sticks offer convenience and precision.
- **Shade Selection**: Choose a contour shade that is two shades darker than your skin tone and a highlighter that is one or two shades lighter. The contour shade should have a cool undertone to mimic natural shadows, while highlighters can range from matte to shimmery based on your preference.

Tools for Application

- **Brushes and Sponges**: Use an angled contour brush for precise application and a fluffy brush for blending powders. A damp makeup sponge is perfect for blending cream products.

Contouring Steps

1. **Prepping the Skin**: Start with a clean, moisturized face and apply your foundation as a base.
2. **Mapping Out Contour Lines**: Using your chosen contour product, draw lines to define the areas you want to recede or slim down. Typical areas include the hollows of your cheeks, sides of the forehead, jawline, and sides of the nose.
3. **Blending**: Blend the contour lines using upward motions for the cheeks and circular motions for the forehead and jawline. The key is to blend thoroughly so there are no harsh lines, creating a subtle shadow effect.

Highlighting Steps

1. **Applying Highlighter**: Apply your highlighter to areas you want to bring forward or emphasize. Common areas include the tops of your cheekbones, the bridge of the nose, the center of the forehead, the cupid's bow, and the chin.
2. **Blending for a Seamless Finish**: Use a clean brush or sponge to blend the highlighter into your skin, ensuring it melds with your base and contour for a natural, radiant finish.

Additional Pro Tips

- **Layering Products**: If using creams, apply them before setting your face with powder. If using powder products, apply them after your foundation has been set.
- **Building Intensity Gradually**: Start with a light hand and build up the product to avoid overdoing it.
- **Symmetry is Key**: Ensure both sides of your face are evenly contoured and highlighted for a balanced look.
- **Setting Your Makeup**: Finish with a setting spray to lock in your contour and highlight, ensuring it lasts all day.

Practice and Patience

- **Experimentation**: Don't hesitate to experiment with different intensities and shades until you find what works best for your face.
- **Learning Curve**: Remember, mastering contouring and highlighting takes time and practice. Each attempt will bring you closer to achieving that perfect, sculpted look.

In essence, contouring and highlighting are about enhancing your natural bone structure and facial features. They're not about altering your appearance, but rather about bringing out the best in your unique beauty. With the right techniques, a little practice, and a lot of blending, you'll be contouring and highlighting like a pro in no time!

Bold Lip Makeup Looks

Embracing a bold lip is like donning a piece of exquisite jewelry – it's a defining element that can elevate your entire makeup look. Bold lips, be it the timeless allure of classic red, the deep sophistication of plum, or the edgy statement of black, are not just about color application; they represent an art form that combines precision, confidence, and self-expression.

Let's delve into the art of perfecting the bold lip, ensuring that each step from preparation to application enhances the beauty of your statement look.

Lip Preparation: Laying the Foundation

- **Exfoliation**: Begin by gently exfoliating your lips. This step removes any flaky skin and provides a smooth canvas. You can use a soft toothbrush or a homemade sugar scrub.
- **Hydration**: Next, hydrate your lips. Apply a nourishing lip balm and let it absorb for a few minutes. Hydrated lips not only look better but also hold onto color longer.

Lip Liner: Defining and Shaping

- **Liner Selection**: Choose a lip liner that closely matches your lipstick. This is crucial for creating a seamless look and preventing color bleeding.
- **Contouring Lips**: Outline your lips with the liner, starting from the cupid's bow and moving outward. If you desire a fuller look, you can slightly overline your natural lip line, but remember, subtlety is key.
- **Filling In**: Fill in your entire lip with the liner. This step creates a color base that helps your lipstick last longer and appear more vibrant.

Lipstick Application: The Main Attraction

- **Applying Lipstick**: Apply your lipstick directly from the tube or use a lip brush for more precision. Start from the center and work your way out.
- **Layering for Longevity**: Blot your lips with a tissue and apply a second layer of lipstick. This technique helps in setting the first layer and extends the wear of your lipstick.

Ensuring Longevity: No Smudge, No Budge

- **Setting with Powder**: For extra staying power, lightly dust translucent powder over your lipstick using a tissue. This sets the color and mattifies any excess shine.
- **Regular Check-ins**: Carry your lipstick for touch-ups, especially after eating or drinking. A bold lip may require maintenance to keep it looking flawless.

Choosing the Right Color: Complementing Your Skin Tone

- **Skin Tone Matching**: Select a shade that flatters your skin tone. Cooler skin tones shine with blue-based reds, while warmer skin tones glow with orange-based reds. Deep plums and blacks are universally flattering but require the confidence to carry them off.
- **Harmony with Makeup**: Ensure your bold lip color harmonizes with the rest of your makeup. With a bold lip, keep the eye and cheek makeup more subdued to let your lips take center stage.

A bold lip is more than just a makeup choice; it's an embodiment of your mood, personality, and style. It speaks volumes about your confidence and willingness to stand out. As you master the art of the bold lip, let your choices reflect your individuality. Whether you're making a statement at a special event or simply want to add a dash of drama to your everyday look, a bold lip can be your signature. So, embrace the boldness, perfect your technique, and let your lips do the talking.

As we conclude Chapter 14: Advanced Techniques - Elevating Your Makeup Mastery, it's my hope that you feel empowered and inspired to explore the vast and vibrant world of advanced makeup. We've journeyed through the intricate and sophisticated realms of iconic makeup styles, and now, it's time to reflect on what we've learned and look forward to how you can apply these new skills in your makeup endeavors.

The smokey eye tutorial opened the door to a world of drama and glamour, showing you how to master this timeless look with confidence. We navigated the nuances of shade selection and blending, emphasizing that the key to a stunning smokey eye lies in the smooth transition of colors. Remember, a smokey eye isn't just a makeup style; it's a statement of elegance and sophistication that you can now create with ease.

In our exploration of contouring and highlighting, we delved into the art of sculpting and defining your facial features. By understanding your unique face shape and mastering the application of contours and highlights, you've learned how to enhance your natural beauty in a subtle yet impactful way. These techniques are not just about transformation; they're about accentuating the beauty that already exists within you.

Finally, our journey into the world of bold lip makeup has equipped you with the skills to make a statement with your lips. From the meticulous preparation of your lips to the careful application of color and ensuring its longevity, you've learned that a bold lip is more than just a choice of shade; it's an expression of your personality and style.

As we close this chapter, I encourage you to take these advanced techniques and make them your own. Makeup is an ever-evolving art form, and you are its artist. Each stroke of your brush, each blend of color, and each choice you make is a reflection of your individuality and creativity. So go ahead, experiment with these new techniques, embrace your unique style, and let your makeup be a reflection of the beautiful person you are.

Thank you for joining me on this journey through advanced makeup techniques. Your dedication to learning and growing in your makeup mastery is commendable. Remember, the world of makeup is limitless, and so are the possibilities for your creativity. Keep practicing, keep experimenting, and above all, keep shining in your own unique way.

Chapter 15: Makeup Hygiene and Maintenance

Welcome to Chapter 15, where we delve into an often overlooked but crucial aspect of makeup artistry - hygiene and maintenance. As you've honed your skills and built your makeup collection, it's vital to remember that the longevity of your products and the health of your skin significantly depend on how well you take care of your tools and cosmetics. In this chapter, we'll cover the essentials of maintaining your makeup and tools, ensuring they remain safe, effective, and in top condition.

Cleaning Your Makeup Tools

As we dive into the essential routine of cleaning your makeup tools, it's important to understand the profound impact it has on both the longevity of your tools and the health of your skin. Regular cleaning of brushes and sponges isn't just a recommended practice; it's a cornerstone of responsible makeup application. Let me guide you through the necessary steps to ensure that your tools are not only clean but also well-maintained, enhancing your makeup experience.

Why Regular Cleaning is a Must

Picture your makeup brushes and sponges as a canvas for your art. Just as a painter wouldn't paint on a dirty canvas, your tools should be pristine to create the perfect look. Brushes and sponges can accumulate bacteria, dead skin cells, and oil, which can lead to skin irritations or even breakouts. Moreover, clean tools are essential for the quality application of products, ensuring that your makeup goes on smoothly and looks its best.

Deep Cleaning: Ensuring Thorough Cleanliness

Deep cleaning your tools should be a regular part of your beauty regimen. Here's how you can do it effectively:

1. **Selecting the Right Cleanser**:
   - For brushes, opt for a gentle brush shampoo or mild hair shampoo. These are formulated to clean without damaging the bristles.
   - For sponges, a cleanser specifically designed for makeup sponges works best, as it's tailored to break down makeup residue efficiently.
2. **The Cleaning Process**:
   - **Brushes**: Hold the brush under lukewarm water to wet the bristles. Apply a small amount of shampoo to your palm and gently swirl the brush in it, working up a lather. Rinse thoroughly, ensuring all the soap and residue are gone.
   - **Sponges**: Submerge your sponge in a bowl of warm, soapy water. Squeeze and knead it to release all the makeup trapped inside. Rinse it until the water runs clear, ensuring all soap is removed.

Daily Cleaning: Quick and Effective

In between deep cleans, it's beneficial to give your tools a quick cleanse, especially if you use them frequently:

- **Quick Cleaning Solution**: A daily brush cleaner spray is an excellent solution for a quick clean. Simply spray it onto the bristles and wipe the brush on a clean towel or paper towel until no more product comes off.

Drying: Preserving the Shape and Integrity

After cleaning, drying your tools correctly is crucial to maintain their shape and function:

1. **Brushes**: Gently squeeze out any excess water from the bristles and reshape them. Lay them flat on a clean towel, allowing air to circulate around them. Avoid standing brushes upright while wet, as water can seep into the handle and loosen the glue over time.
2. **Sponges**: Squeeze out the excess water and set them on a clean towel in a well-ventilated area. Ensure they are completely dry before your next use.

By incorporating these cleaning and drying techniques into your routine, you not only safeguard your skin against potential irritants but also extend the life and efficacy of your beloved makeup tools. Remember, in the world of makeup, cleanliness is as important as creativity. So, embrace this essential aspect of your makeup journey, and let the cleanliness of your tools reflect the artistry of your work.

When to Replace Makeup Products

In the captivating journey of makeup artistry, it's essential to recognize that every product in your arsenal has its own lifespan, much like the characters in a story. As we turn the page to the topic of when to replace makeup products, it's crucial to understand that this isn't just about getting the most out of your makeup; it's about safeguarding your skin's health and ensuring the best possible application.

Understanding the Shelf Life of Makeup Products

Each makeup item, from the mascara that accentuates your eyes to the foundation that creates a flawless base, comes with a specific shelf life. This lifespan is a guideline for when a product should ideally be replaced to maintain its effectiveness and hygiene.

1. **Mascara and Liquid Eyeliner**: These are often the shortest-lived in your makeup bag, typically lasting about 3-6 months. Due to their liquid nature and proximity to your eyes, they're prone to bacterial buildup.
2. **Lipsticks and Lip Glosses**: Generally, these can last up to a year, but if you notice a change in texture or smell, it's time to bid them farewell.

3. **Foundations and Concealers**: Water-based versions tend to last up to a year, while oil-based formulas can stretch a bit longer.
4. **Powders**: Powder-based products like blushes, eyeshadows, and setting powders have a longer shelf life, often up to two years.

Spotting the Signs of Expiration

Like a skilled detective, learn to spot the clues that indicate a makeup product is past its prime:

- **Texture Changes**: If a product changes in consistency – for instance, if a lipstick gets too hard or a liquid foundation separates – it's a sign that it's time to replace it.
- **Odor**: Any change in smell is a clear indicator that a product should no longer be used.
- **Performance**: If the product doesn't apply or blend as it once did, it might be time to let it go.

The Risks of Using Expired Makeup

Using expired makeup isn't just a minor faux pas; it can pose real risks to your skin and eyes:

- **Skin Irritations**: Expired products can lead to skin irritations, breakouts, and allergic reactions.
- **Eye Infections**: Old mascara and eyeliners are particularly notorious for causing eye infections.

Embracing Product Replacement

While it might be hard to part with your favorite blush or lipstick, replacing your makeup regularly is a necessary ritual in your beauty routine. It ensures that what you're putting on your skin is safe, effective, and performs as it should.

Remember, your makeup collection is a dynamic ensemble, ever-evolving with products coming and going. By staying vigilant about the shelf life and condition of your makeup, you're not just taking care of your products; you're taking care of yourself. Keep this guide in mind as you curate your collection, and let the practice of timely replacement be a testament to your commitment to both beauty and well-being.

Storing Your Makeup Correctly

Just as a painter cherishes their brushes and paints, storing your makeup correctly is pivotal in preserving the life and quality of your beloved beauty products. Proper storage isn't just about tidiness; it's about extending the lifespan of your makeup and ensuring its best performance. Let's explore the art of storing your makeup, from the cozy confines of your vanity to the adventures of travel.

Mastering the Art of Proper Makeup Storage

Think of your makeup as delicate treasures, each requiring its own special care. The way you store them can significantly impact their longevity and efficacy.

1. **Understanding the Environment**: Makeup's worst enemies include extreme temperatures, humidity, and direct sunlight. These factors can degrade the quality and shorten the lifespan of your products. For example, excessive heat can cause creams and lipsticks to melt, while humidity can encourage bacterial growth in products.
2. **The Ideal Setting**: Aim to store your makeup in a cool, dry place away from direct sunlight. A bedroom vanity or a bathroom cabinet (if it's not too steamy) can be perfect spots.

Organizing Your Makeup Collection

An organized makeup collection is not just aesthetically pleasing but also functional in maintaining the quality of your products.

- **Separation is Key**: Keep your daily-use products within easy reach, while more occasional items can be stored away.
- **Use Organizers**: Drawer dividers, makeup holders, and storage boxes can be invaluable in keeping your products organized and easily accessible.
- **Regular Inventory**: Periodically go through your collection. This not only helps in keeping it organized but also allows you to check on the condition of your products and discard any that are expired or damaged.

Travel Tips: Taking Your Makeup on the Road

For those who love to travel, keeping your makeup safe and hygienic while on the move is essential.

1. **Choosing the Right Bag**: Opt for a makeup bag that is spacious enough to hold your essentials but compact enough to fit in your luggage. Look for one with compartments to keep products separate and secure.
2. **Protection is Crucial**: For fragile items like powder compacts, consider additional cushioning. Bubble wrap or padded pouches can prevent breakage.
3. **Avoiding Leaks**: For liquid products, tighten the lids and consider sealing them in ziplock bags to prevent any messy leaks.
4. **Hygiene First**: Regularly clean your makeup bag to keep it hygienic and free from product residue or spills.

By adopting these storage and organization practices, you're not just tidying up; you're ensuring that each product remains in its optimal state, ready to perform when you need it. A well-organized makeup collection is a canvas for your creativity, where every product is cared for and every choice is an informed one.

So, embrace these storage strategies, and let your makeup collection be a reflection of both your beauty and your meticulous care. With your products neatly stored and organized, you're ready to create beauty, whether at home or on the go.

By the end of this chapter, you'll be equipped with the knowledge and techniques to maintain a hygienic and well-organized makeup collection. Remember, good hygiene practices in makeup are not just about cleanliness; they're an integral part of being a responsible and skilled makeup enthusiast. Let's embark on this journey to ensure the longevity of your beloved products and the health of your skin.

Chapter 16: Ethical and Sustainable Makeup Choices

In the world of beauty and cosmetics, there's a growing awareness about the impact our choices have on the environment and on animal welfare. Chapter 16 is dedicated to navigating the realms of ethical and sustainable makeup. Here, we'll dive deep into understanding what it means to choose cruelty-free and vegan products, the importance of eco-friendly brands, and how to make responsible makeup choices that align with a conscientious lifestyle.

Understanding Cruelty-Free and Vegan Makeup

- **Cruelty-Free Products**: These products are developed without any form of animal testing at any stage of their production. This practice not only concerns the final product but also its ingredients. The certification process for cruelty-free products involves rigorous checks to ensure that no animal testing is used.
- **Vegan Makeup**: Vegan makeup takes ethical considerations a step further by ensuring no animal-derived ingredients are present in the products. Common non-vegan ingredients in makeup include beeswax, lanolin, collagen, and keratin. Opting for vegan makeup is a choice that supports animal welfare and often leads to products that are gentler on the skin.
- **How to Identify**: Look for certifications like the Leaping Bunny, PETA's cruelty-free logo, or the Vegan Society trademark. These symbols on your makeup products assure that they meet the strict standards of being cruelty-free or vegan.

Eco-Friendly Makeup Brands and Products

- **Sustainable Practices**: Some makeup brands focus on sustainability by implementing eco-friendly practices in manufacturing, packaging, and ingredient sourcing. They often use organic and natural ingredients, ensuring that their products are free from harmful chemicals and environmentally damaging substances.
- **Environmentally Conscious Packaging**: These brands might use recycled materials for packaging, implement refillable systems, or design products with minimal packaging to reduce waste.
- **Notable Eco-Friendly Brands**: Brands like Ilia, RMS Beauty, and Aether Beauty are known for their commitment to sustainability and eco-conscious practices. They offer a range of products that are both beautiful and kind to the planet.

Making Responsible Makeup Choices

- **Conscious Consumerism**: Being a conscious consumer involves more than just buying products; it's about understanding the entire lifecycle of your makeup, from production to disposal. It means choosing products that are not only good for you but also for the environment.
- **Reducing Waste**: You can reduce waste by choosing products with less packaging, opting for refillable options, and properly recycling your makeup containers once they're empty.
- **DIY Makeup Options**: For those interested in a hands-on approach, creating your own makeup can be a sustainable alternative. Homemade makeup allows you to control the ingredients, reducing the environmental impact and avoiding unnecessary packaging.
- **Educating and Spreading Awareness**: Informed choices come from being well-educated. Learning about the environmental and ethical impacts of makeup and sharing this knowledge can lead to a wider impact and encourage others to make responsible choices.

Through this chapter, we aim to shed light on the importance of ethical and sustainable practices in the beauty industry. By making informed choices, you contribute to a movement that values our planet and its inhabitants, ensuring that the beauty world is not just about looking good, but also about doing good.

Conclusion: Embracing Your Makeup Journey

As we reach the conclusion of this comprehensive guide to makeup artistry, it's an opportune moment to pause and reflect on the transformative journey we've taken. From the fundamental basics to the intricate details of advanced techniques, this guide has aimed to unveil the full spectrum of makeup's potential. It's a journey that has highlighted the power of makeup not just as a tool for aesthetic enhancement, but as a medium for personal expression and creativity. Let's revisit the key milestones of this journey, celebrate the skills you've acquired, and look forward to the continued evolution of your personal makeup artistry.

Recap of Key Makeup Skills

- **Mastering the Basics**: We embarked on this journey by laying a solid foundation, exploring the intricacies of skin types, familiarizing ourselves with essential makeup tools, and mastering the application of foundational products like foundation, concealer, and setting powders. These foundational skills form the cornerstone of any successful makeup application, providing the groundwork upon which all other techniques are built.
- **Eye Makeup Mastery**: We navigated the art of eye makeup, delving into techniques ranging from the subtlety of everyday looks to the dramatic flair of smokey eyes and winged liners. You've learned how to enhance and accentuate the eyes, a central feature of expression in makeup artistry.
- **Lip Artistry**: The journey also took us through the colorful world of lip makeup. Here, you've gained insight into selecting the right shades for your skin tone, applying lip products with precision, and making bold statements with striking lip colors.
- **Advanced Makeup Techniques**: As your skills progressed, we ventured into more advanced territories like contouring, highlighting, and crafting specific makeup styles. These techniques have empowered you to elevate your makeup artistry, adding depth, dimension, and sophistication to your creations.
- **Ethical and Sustainable Makeup Choices**: In recognizing the broader impact of our makeup choices, we explored the importance of ethical and sustainable practices in the beauty industry. This awareness enables you to make choices that are not only beautiful but also kind and considerate to our planet and its inhabitants.

Encouragement for Your Personal Makeup Journey

- **The Beauty of Continuous Learning**: The world of makeup is ever-evolving, with new trends, products, and techniques continually emerging. Embrace this journey with a spirit of curiosity and a willingness to keep learning and growing.
- **Personal Style and Expression**: Remember, makeup is a form of personal artistry. Let it reflect who you are, your mood, and your individual style. There's a unique beauty in how makeup can be adapted to express different facets of your personality.

- **Creativity and Experimentation**: Don't shy away from experimentation. Trying new colors, mixing products, and exploring various styles are integral to discovering what resonates with you. It's through experimentation that your unique makeup style will flourish.
- **Building Community and Sharing Knowledge**: The beauty community is rich with inspiration and learning. Engage with fellow makeup enthusiasts, share your experiences, and draw inspiration from the collective creativity and knowledge of the community.
- **Prioritizing Health and Wellness**: Above all, makeup should complement your overall wellness. Choose products that harmonize with your skin type and contribute positively to your skin's health. Remember, true beauty stems from both internal and external well-being.

As this guide concludes, remember that it represents just one chapter in the ongoing narrative of your makeup journey. Armed with brushes and a palette of endless possibilities, step forward with confidence and joy. Embrace your newfound skills, cherish your individuality, and let your inner beauty radiate. Here's to the beautiful moments, the transformative experiences, and the endless creativity that awaits you in the vibrant and ever-changing world of makeup!